From Backpack
to Briefcase

From Backpack to Briefcase

PROFESSIONAL DEVELOPMENT IN HEALTH CARE ADMINISTRATION

Michael R. Meacham JD, MPH

Medical University of South Carolina

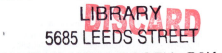
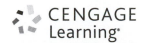

CENGAGE
Learning·

Australia · Brazil · Mexico · Singapore · United Kingdom · United States

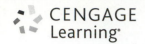

**From Backpack to Briefcase:
Professional Development in
Health Care Administration**
Michael R. Meacham JD, MPH

Senior Vice President, GM Skills & Product Planning: Dawn Gerrain

Product Manager: Jadin B. Kavanaugh

Senior Director, Development-Career and Computing: Marah Bellegarde

Product Development Manager: Juliet Steiner

Marketing Director: Michele McTighe

Marketing Manager: Erica Glisson

Senior Production Director: Wendy Troeger

Production Manager: Andrew Crouth

Content Project Management and Art Direction: Lumina Datamatics, Inc.

Cover image(s): Businessman signing a document: © iStockphoto.com/ Neustockimages; African-American college

Graduate: © iStockphoto.com/kickstand; close-up of businessman hand holding briefcase: © Pressmaster/Shutterstock

Library of Congress Control Number: 2014937120

ISBN: 978-1-285-08485-5

Cengage Learning
20 Channel Center Street
Boston, MA 02210
USA

Cengage Learning is a leading provider of customized learning solutions with office locations around the globe, including Singapore, the United Kingdom, Australia, Mexico, Brazil, and Japan. Locate your local office at: **www.cengage.com/global**

Cengage Learning products are represented in Canada by Nelson Education, Ltd.

To learn more about Cengage Learning, visit **www.cengage.com**

Purchase any of our products at your local college store or at our preferred online store **www.cengagebrain.com**

Printed in the United States of America
Print Number: 01   Print Year: 2014

DEDICATION

For the love of my life, my wife, and best friend, Vicky Triponey

TABLE OF CONTENTS

CONTRIBUTORS

Jessica Boss
Pharmaceutical Sales Representative for
Jazz Pharmaceuticals
Los Angeles, CA

Sarah Boyd
Owner of SJBusiness Partners, LLC
Charleston, SC

Donald Brunn, MHSA, FACHE
President and Chief Operating Officer of
The Emory Clinic
Atlanta, GA

Bill Burmeister
Business Operations Manager Middlesex Hospital
Middlesex, CT

Gayle L. Capozzallo, FACHE
COO Yale-New Haven Health System
Chairperson, American College of Healthcare
Executives (2012–2013)
New Haven, CT

Tom Charles
Senior Vice President for System Development and
Chief Strategy Officer for Mount Nittany Health
State College, PA

Kyle Dorsey
Health Center Administrator Advanced Heart and
Lung Failure
Duke University Medical Center
Durham, NC

Emily Hardeman
Associate Project Director in the Office of the Senior
Vice President and Chief of Clinical Operations
at The University of Texas MD Anderson Cancer
Center
Houston, TX

Cindy Helling
Executive Director, Select Health of South Carolina
Charleston, SC

Jeffery Knorr
Administrative Director for Women's Health Services
for the University of Pittsburgh Medical Center
physician practices
Pittsburgh, PA

Laura F. Leahy, MHA
Practice Manager of Internal Medicine and Immediate
Care at Northwestern Memorial Physicians Group
Chicago, IL

Jill Pletcher
Director of Career Services at Wichita State University
Wichita, KS

Jacque Richardson
Executive Director, The Lakes at Litchfield
Pawleys Island, SC

Diane Simmons, MPA RN CAE
Vice President, Education and Certification with the
Healthcare Financial Management Association
Chicago, IL

Anthony C. Stanowski, FACHE
Vice President—Applied Medical Software
Collingswood, NJ

Steven Wagman
Vice President for Enterprise Solutions Implementation
at Siemens Medical Solutions, USA
Malvern, PA

PREFACE

From Backpack to Briefcase: Professional Development in Health Administration

This book is intended to help both undergraduate students of health administration as well as Master of Health Administration students as they move from classroom to internship or from campus to career professional. There are plenty of books in the market that tell you how to write a resume. There are none, however, that speak to health administration students regarding the state of the industry and how to look for one of the many career paths in the multifaceted industry we call "health services."

This book will help students prepare for the internship or job search by improving their understanding of who they are and why they are interested in health care. By focusing on those foundational questions, it becomes a bit easier, then, to write the cover letter expressing an interest in one aspect or another of the health care business. This book is for those students, who once having undertaken that additional step of self-discovery, then want to learn more about the practical steps of career development: constructing a resume to create a snap shot of their accumulated experiences; conducting a phone or Skype interview to get to the next step; how to handle some of the intensity of the on-site interview; what to do after each of these phases in the job search; and so forth.

But beyond that, this book also speaks to those young professionals emerging from undergraduate and MHA programs who are preparing to move into their first professional positions: how to dress; how to handle what seems to be the endless stream of meetings; how to understand that no job is too small; and that the first job is to help the boss look good.

The reason for the book is pretty simple. The number of both undergraduate and MHA programs is growing. The number of students enrolled in both undergraduate and MHA programs is also growing. As faculty, we see an increasing need for "professional development" among students who come to the programs with insufficient tools to relate to the professional world. At the same time, there are no textbooks that speak to the specific needs of health administration students to help them bridge the divide from classroom to workplace; to help them translate the culture of backpack to briefcase.

ORGANIZATION

The text begins with some introspection to help the student discover more about themselves in order that they might see the world around them with a bit more clarity. In Chapter 1, students are asked to consider their own values and who their heroes and heroines are. They are also asked to deeply consider what they want to get from life and how they will know when they get it. This understanding is helpful as they think about why they are in health care and what role they want to play in it.

From that "internal" perspective, the text then takes the student to an "external" perspective in Chapter 2. How do they look and sound in the eyes and ears of others, reminding them that everyone they meet is a potential reference, network contact, employer, or other valuable asset in their professional world. Thus, their appearance and demeanor are important in supporting the role and goal they have referenced in the first response. The use—and misuse—of social media is included in this discussion.

Chapter 3 provides a discussion about researching to find the right kind of employer. Again, drawing on the inner strength and values emanating from the first response, students will more naturally be able to gravitate to responses to this kind of research.

Next, Chapter 4 covers the importance of professional networking, what it is, how to do it, where it takes place, and why it is important.

Chapter 5 is about the cover letter: how to match the stationery and the letterhead to the resume; how to write the cover letter; how circumstances will change the content and structure of the letter; and what to do about the electronic application. Examples of cover letters are provided.

As one might expect, the next item in the logical sequence would be a chapter on the resume. In Chapter 6 examples are provided, highlighting both *dos* and *don'ts* for the reader to see clearly how a good resume is assembled. A table of action verbs is included along with a discussion about why using action verbs is important.

Chapter 7 deals with the preliminary interviews—telephone interviews and Skype interviews. The student will learn how to diplomatically ask for additional information; how to relate with the prospective employer's staff; learn some of the more likely types of questions they might encounter and what to do both before the interview actually takes place; and what to do when it is over.

Chapter 8 goes into a good bit of detail regarding the on-site interview, discussing types of questions that may be covered, questions the student may wish to ask or consider, the finer points of the "interview meal," and some tips about evaluating a job offer, including salary and benefits.

Chapters 9 and 10 are dedicated to the notion of the ethics of accepting a job offer, the concept of "fit," and how you make the most of it once you are there. These chapters discuss the need for lifelong learning, the need to give back to the profession, the importance about the concept of service to the organization, the importance about projects and mentors, as well as a discussion about e-mail etiquette.

A final note about how the chapters are organized. Throughout the first 10 chapters are sidebars written by industry professionals that speak to a key subject pertinent to that chapter from the professional's perspective. Thus, the former Chairperson of the ACHE Board, Gayle Capozollo of Yale-New Haven Hospital, writes about the importance of giving back to the profession in chapter 9; Don Brunn of Emory Health care writes about what they look for in a management development candidate in Chapter 7. The professionals dispense outstanding advice throughout the first 10 chapters of the book.

The 11th chapter is a compendium of essays from a variety of professional administrators writing about "A Day in the Life of. . . ." From primary care practice administrators to pharmaceutical sales representatives to imaging technology executives—along with a host of others—students will be able to sample vicariously the lives of health care executives from a wide variety of perspectives.

There are exercises throughout the book that will help the student apply the material from the chapters. Often these involve a partner, because sometimes the best way we can learn about ourselves is through the eyes of another.

The result should be a comprehensive text that takes the student symbolically, if not in fact, from the popular backpack used on campus to the briefcase one might use to carry one's "homework" to and from the office as a professional. Enjoy the journey!

FEATURES

Key elements of the text to support student understanding of these topics include:

- Sidebars that provide expert observation and commentary, enriching the chapter with additional detail.
- Photos to give realistic visual examples of references in the text.
- Conclusions that briefly encapsulate the most important "take away" points of the chapter.
- Exercises for self-development give the student an opportunity to prepare the documents they will need for a successful job search.

ABOUT THE AUTHOR

Michael R. Meacham, J.D. (*University of Kansas*), **M.P.H.** (*University of Kansas School of Medicine/ Wichita State University*), **Associate Professor.** Mr. Meacham has an extensive background in development, enactment, and implementation of public policy as well as in leadership and management of healthcare organizations. He served eight years in the Kansas House of Representatives, having been elected while a law student in 1976, two years after his graduation from Wichita State University. In 1998, Mr. Meacham left his legal practice in Kansas to become Director of Health System Development for Connecticut's Office of Health Care Access where he led administrative improvements in that state's Certificate of Need Law and other regulatory reforms affecting health services organizations. In March 2001, Mr. Meacham was named Vice President for Integrated Health Services at Eastern Connecticut Health Network, with responsibility for multiple healthcare units, including administrative and clinical personnel, leading the successful implementation of a two-campus hospitalist system, in addition to other responsibilities. He was named an Associate Professor at Pennsylvania State University in July 2003. As an instructor and as a student of health care, Mr. Meacham's interests are in strategic planning for health care organizations, management, leadership, health policy, and predominately with the development of students as young professionals. Mr. Meacham joined the Medical University of South Carolina faculty in July 2010 as Associate Professor of Health Leadership and Management where he teaches in both the Doctor of Health Administration and the Master of Health Administration programs. Because of his close work with students in professional development, Mr. Meacham was nominated for MUSC Foundation's 2014 *Teaching Excellence Award* in the *Educator-Mentor: Clinical Professional* Category.

ACKNOWLEDGMENTS

No one accomplishes writing a book alone, though the act of writing itself seems like a form of solitary confinement at times. In the end, however, there are many people who help. For me there were two very special people at the top of the list. As I wrote the book, I thought it would be interesting and informative to have feedback from people who would actually be using it. So as I wrote each chapter I asked two students to review and provide feedback. I am deeply indebted to Medical University of South Carolina MHA student (and now alum) Janna Cone and former Western Kentucky University undergraduate student (and current Medical University of South Carolina MHA student) Paige Montgomery for the many hours they devoted to reading chapter by chapter and providing detailed commentary that was insightful and wise in helping me shape the ultimate product. The book is much better as a result of their contributions.

Likewise, as the book goes through the publication process, the audience that actually makes the decision to use—or not use—the book also reviews the text. In this vein, I am deeply indebted to Matt Brooks of Texas State University, Andy Garman CEO of the National Center for Healthcare Leadership and Professor at Rush University, Randa Hall of University of Alabama at Birmingham, Diane Howard of Rush University, Christy Harris Lemak of University of Alabama at—Birmingham and Jon Thompson of James Madison University. I also want to thank Barb Pultorak who did an initial copy review and edit for me.

Finally, but certainly not least, I would like to express my appreciation to all the people at Cengage Learning who helped bring this concept to life, most especially Juliet Steiner who came to the project at a critical time and provided essential leadership and support in getting it across the finish line "on time and on budget" as they say.

REVIEWERS

Matthew S. Brooks, PhD, FACHE, CPH
Associate Professor and Director School of Health
   Administration
College of Health Professions
Texas State University
San Marcos, TX

Andy Garman, PsyD
Professor and Chief Executive Officer
National Center for Healthcare Leadership
College of Health Sciences
Rush University

Randa S. Hall, MBA
Master of Science in Health Administration Program
   Director
Department of Health Services Administration
School of Health Professions
University of Alabama at Birmingham
Birmingham, AL

Diane M. Howard, PhD, FACHE
Director of Student Development and Assistant
   Professor Department of Health Systems
   Management
College of Health Sciences
Rush University
Chicago, IL

Christy Harris Lemak, PhD, FACHE
Department Chair
Department of Health Services Administration
School of Health Professions
University of Alabama at Birmingham

Jon M. Thompson, PhD
Professor and Director Health Services Administration
   Program
Department of Health Sciences
College of Health and Behavioral Studies
James Madison University
Harrisonburg, VA

STUDENT REVIEWERS

Janna Cone, MHA
Medical University of South Carolina
Charleston, SC

Paige Montgomery, BA
Western Kentucky University
Bowling Green, KY

Discovering Who You Are: How Do You Explain to an Employer Who You Are If You Do Not Know Yourself?

PROFESSIONAL DEVELOPMENT

What does *that* mean? To be a professional means providing a service to others. Furthermore, it means serving others with an idea that the principle end result is not really about money, but rather about rendering a service that has meaning to those who receive it. Of course, a professional is to be compensated, but the *primary* objective is to provide a service that benefits another, not improving a profit margin. The third element of being a professional is that the service should not only be of benefit to an individual, but should be a service that is beneficial to society as a whole.

You have chosen a career in health care administration—a profession that provides a service by organizing increasingly precious resources to provide the best quality of care available at the least possible cost to the maximum number of people who can feasibly be served. Does that sound like it intends to benefit both individuals and society? It should because that *is* the mission. Do we sometimes miss the mark? Of course, we do. That does not mean we do not believe in or abandon the mission. Oh yes, about the money part: Few of us are overpaid. Admittedly, there are sometimes abuses that occur in a handful of organizations near or at the very top, but given the number of health

care organizations in the United States that would seem to be a very small percentage of the time.

For you, *professional* means to organize, manage, and distribute limited health care resources in our communities to effectively benefit as many people as we possibly can at the lowest feasible cost.

Development is the second part of the term that we need to define. You do not simply show up one day and pronounce "I, the 'professional' have arrived!" There are certain things you need to know to fully function on the professional level to which you aspire. To be clear, these include certain aspects of accounting, finance, statistics, management, quality of care, strategy, human resources, epidemiology, marketing, reimbursement, and other subsets of health care administration. Those are the real substantive areas of health care administration and, indeed, the real substantive areas of *professional development*. For our purposes, however, *professional development* will speak more to the inner you as well as to the stylistic pieces of being professional. You can know everything there is to know about running a major health services organization, but you will have no credibility if you walk around in dirty jeans, last week's T-shirt, flip-flops, and a five-day old beard. OK, that might be a bit extreme, but you get the picture. Likewise, however, you can have the same knowledge, be "dressed to the nines," but if you do not have what it takes to speak up at the appropriate time in the meetings, you will be fundamentally shut out of the decision-making process and the organization will have missed out on engaging one of its best resources. Professional development then, for the purposes of this book, is about a journey of self-discovery and self-reflection in order to better adapt your skill set to the world around you and is also about how to make an impressive outward appearance, so you can make an opportunity for yourself to apply what you know and move your career forward.

Professional development can only begin in one place, and that is with you. It is about understanding *who* you are; *how* you came to be here; *why* you are here; and *what* you want to achieve. Now for the hard part: No one can tell you the answers to any of these questions. The answers to who you are, what you are, and why you are on this earth can only be determined and articulated by you.

You will not find it in a book chapter; your professor cannot give you a lecture and PowerPoint with the answers. Above all, you will *not* be able to go to the web and find the answer. Google cannot help you with this one. (See Figure 1-1.)

How you answer these questions forms your overall self-impression. Your self-impression means a great deal; in many instances, how you see yourself will be how others see you. There is an anonymous old saying: "Value yourself highly, because the world takes you at your own estimate." Employers are looking for people who have certain demonstrated skills and who will be able to work well with others, because virtually nothing about health care management is accomplished by working alone. As a result, employers will want to know about *you*, so it is foundational to be able to answer questions about yourself. And not just for employers, but for yourself as well. As you become more self-aware, you will find that you *fit* better in some circumstances than others. *That* is perfectly OK. Indeed, one of the things discussed later in this book is the notion of having a "fit" with an employer. You do not need to take the first job that comes along; you do not need to take just "any" job. You have the right to be in an environment that will be professionally challenging

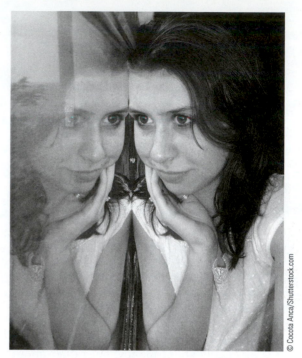

Figure 1-1 Who am I? Understanding one's self is a first step toward professional development.

and rewarding—one where you can make a positive contribution and feel a sense of achievement for it. This is what *value yourself highly* means. It is not about a sense of "I'm better than anyone else," but about understanding that you have the power to determine your identity. And that includes the power to choose a work environment that is well-suited, not only to your skills, but also to your sense of values, your sense about who you are. The catch is that you will not know what such a place is like without first understanding more about yourself.

This chapter will present you with a series of exercises about you. Expect to be uncomfortable—self-assessment and introspection are almost always uncomfortable. This chapter will focus on four different elements of you: (1) knowing who you are; (2) understanding your unique qualities; (3) defining the purpose of your life; and (4) answering the following question: "Why do I want to be in health care?" There will be exercises about each of these elements, preceded by introductory comments.

DESCRIBING YOURSELF

A host of things comprises who we are. (Genetic composition, as we know, is critically important, but as we cannot do anything about that, we will focus on environmental factors.) This section will help you discover something *about how where* and *who* have contributed to your growth and development to this point in your life.

Where Am I From?

Our environment plays an enormous role in defining who we are. Are you from the farm or the big city? Or perhaps from suburbia? What kinds of jobs do/did your parents have? Are you the first from your family to go to college? To graduate from college? Or are you a third generation legacy at your state's flagship university? Are you poor, middle class, or wealthy? Are you Caucasian, Hispanic, African-American, Asian-American, or of mixed race? Is your family a happy and supportive one? Or have you had to achieve in spite of negative attitudes from some family members? All of these things, and more, describe where we are from.

How Does Where I Am from Influence Me?

People will look at the world in a different way depending on how and where they grew up. To paint the obvious example, the person who grew up white, lived in affluent suburbia, attended private schools, and had parents who supported (but not doted) is likely to see the world in a lot different light than the person who grew up black, lived in an inner city housing project, who attended an under-resourced public school, and had only one parent who wished their child would work instead of going to school. Those are two vastly different worlds; and the people who grew up in them will probably see the world in entirely different ways as a result. One may grow up with a sense of entitlement—that the world is already his and that he merely needs to show up to get the prize, whatever it may be. Similarly, the other person may develop a strong will to succeed along with a work ethic that incorporates the concept that

no project is too small a foundation upon which to build. Likewise, growing up in an urban area will create a different view of the world than growing up in a small town or out on the farm. You may have heard the expression that "How you view something depends on where you sit." How you look at the world does indeed depend largely on the part of it in which you have grown up.

What Are My Values?

This gets us to the core pretty quickly. Are you the kind of person who wants to get ahead by demonstrating effective problem solving; who does not cheat on tests; or who reads the assigned material? Or are you the person who understands that you can take a short-cut now and again; who can work collaboratively with someone on an assignment that is intended to be your work alone; or who captures material from the web to use in place of original thought? Are there moral absolutes for you? Or are things relative? Are you interested in a "common good," or is it "every person for themself" for you? Chapter 9 will delve more deeply into the topic of ethics, but the message begins here: Health care is not easy; patients entrust themselves to our care at times in their lives in which they are vulnerable and sometimes confronting grave circumstances. Our job is to *serve* them and we cannot do that job competently if our core values are constructed in such a way as to devalue the human experience by ignoring ethical and professional concepts. If your values are "situational," then perhaps another line of work might be more appropriate for you. If you believe in the concept of *sustainable* values, what we *should* and *should not* be doing, then health care might be a good fit for you.

Who Influences You?

To whom do you listen for advice? Do you seek out people who have "been around the block a few times" who have life experiences to share? Or do you discuss things with peers and let them help you guide your judgments? Do you find subject matter experts? Do you find strength in prayer? Do you have a mentor on whom you rely for wisdom? Who is it that helps you understand the world and, thereby, influences you?

Many of us have been fortunate enough to have a mentor in our lives. Some people may have had several mentors throughout several phases of their academic and professional careers. Those are the people who help shape us by teaching us the things that are not between the covers of a textbook or the things that are not glowing from an e-reader. Mentors teach many things. Some can help with writing skills, perhaps like what is happening in Figure 1-2, while others may help with other interpersonal skills.

What Influences You?

Obviously, we have all been influenced by significant events. Every generation has *the moment* that *everyone* remembers where they were when it happened. Those events remain seared into our memories. And other events, even though not so traumatic, also help shape us and influence us. For some it is the experience of being on an athletic team and learning to understand the concept of teamwork; for others it is the joy of discovery when the eighth grade science experiment works. In addition to events, however, should be the "what else." The "what else" should, of course, be elements of your commitment to lifelong learning. This is another way of saying that books, journals, newspapers, and magazines, even the electronic versions of them, are things you should be reading and they should be influencing you because of the new knowledge you acquire from them. I was deeply influenced early

in my health care career by Paul Starr's *The Social Transformation of American Medicine* and there is not a semester, probably not a month, that goes by without my recommending it to someone (Starr, 1982). In the words of Oliver Wendell Holmes, Jr. "A mind once stretched by a new idea never regains its original dimension" (Holmes, n.d.).

Who Do You Admire?

Who are your heroes and heroines? Are they political? Are they in business? Are they religious leaders? If you could model yourself after someone, who would it be? Why? Think about those individuals in depth. Why are they your heroes/heroines? What is it about their achievement that stands out in your mind?

What Is Important to You?

Do you value family or are you more interested in a career? Do you care about having a *balance* in work and family life, or are you driven to succeed? Or are you willing to sacrifice career achievement to have a terrific family life? Is money what drives you? Or is it service to some cause greater than self?

These are the basic elements of "who you are." We are, genetic characteristics aside, the sum of our experiences. Experiences have created certain lessons for all of us. What is good or bad? What makes us happy? What gives us a sense of achievement? What causes us to be stressed? Life environments, the people we care about and admire, our values, all comprise "who you are."

UNDERSTANDING YOUR UNIQUE QUALITIES

Each of us has unique qualities. Aside from color of hair or eyes, or other physical attributes, each of us has a way of doing things, when taken in combination, makes us genuinely unique individuals. To assess those qualities we will discuss particular skills you may possess, the method you use to achieve, where you sense you belong, and what you can contribute.

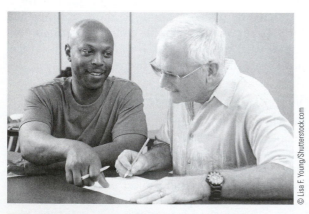

© Lisa F. Young/Shutterstock.com

Figure 1-2 A mentor helping a student.

LOOKING BEYOND SELF: A BRIEF DISCUSSION ABOUT DIVERSITY

While this chapter—and indeed the entire book—is about *you*, it would be incomplete if it did not encourage you to also reflect about you in the context of the larger world. As a society, we are becoming increasingly diverse, and as that occurs, it will change the way we communicate with colleagues and patients; it will change the composition of both the workforce and the patient population. And it will present both challenges and opportunities about how we do our work and conduct our lives.

To give you an idea about just how rapidly our population is changing, consider this: In 1950, census data indicted 89.3% of the American population was Caucasian (in those days "white") and only 9.9% African-American (in those days "black") with just 0.7% coming from *all* other groups. Persons of Hispanic or Latino origins were not counted separately at that time (Bureau of the Census, 1980). By 1980, the population broke down along these ethnic lines: Caucasian 83.1%; African-American 11.7%; Hispanic or Latino origin 6.4%; Asian-American 1.5%; and other 3.6% (Bureau of the Census, 1980). Just in the span of 30 years the American population had become so diverse that the Census Bureau had to increase its level of detail and sophistication to capture the data and report the population statistics. From that we see substantial growth in the three largest non-Caucasian ethnic groups. But this trend is not linear; it is exponential. Thus, 2012 census data reported the following composition in the U.S. population: Caucasian 63%; Hispanic or Latino origins 16.9%; African-American 13.1%; Asian-American 5.3%; and other 1.7% (Bureau of the Census, 2013). As you can see, the growth of all the ethnic groups relative to the Caucasian population has been dramatic.

Not only are we becoming more ethnically diverse, but we are aging as well. The baby boomer population began easing into retirement in 2010 at the rate of 10,000 per day. What this means is that the population for which you will provide care will be both dramatically more diverse and considerably older. In 2010, 13% of the population was over 65. By the time you are in the prime of your career, 2050, one in five Americans will be over 65 years of age (Bureau of the Census, 1994). This has enormous implications for service demands as well as payment for services. To compound the situation, this generation will be extraordinarily well informed as health consumers and unrelenting in demanding more and better care.

But *diversity* means much more than age and race. It includes cultural differences, religious differences, gender, sexual identity and sexual orientation, as well as heritage. Also included are things like educational attainment, parental status, and geographic location. Virtually, all of these elements are changing; there are more children in unmarried households; we have attained the highest level of education in U.S. history; and we have a greater awareness of differences surrounding sexuality. All of this has implications for leadership and patient care. We—and our colleagues on the front lines of care—will need to be much more culturally aware and sensitive. While this may present some challenges, the opportunities are much more significant. As we embrace—not merely tolerate—our differences, we will find we are stronger as a culture and as a nation. As we include ideas from other perspectives about problem solving, we will find we are more creative and will engage ideas we have not yet considered, thereby making for stronger management teams. Those organizations that proactively embrace and foster diversity in the workplace will find not only are they more creative, but they will become the employer of choice in their respective communities. In addition, patients will be more comfortable in their care than in an organization that remains mired in the traditions of the past.

(continues)

(continued)

From an individual perspective, this note is here because it is important that you see the direction of our culture and embrace it. Just 60 years ago, as a population, the United States was basically 90% white and 10% black; today, it is approximately 2/3 Caucasian with the other 1/3 of multiple origins and races. And 60 years from today—still within the span of your lifetime, the U.S. population will be even more diverse. Your success, in no small measure, will depend on your ability to forge relationships with people from vastly different backgrounds than yours. We are a wide mix of people on this planet. We know that virtually everything, including health care, is becoming increasingly global. Among other implications, globalization means the rate of change will likely accelerate. As that occurs, those who recognize that we are all connected to one another in some way and seek to find common understandings with those who are "different" from us will become transformational leaders. Those who eschew others who do not look like themselves will find they are at an increasing professional disadvantage and living with the absence of social enrichment that comes through associations with others. While the exercises here are intended to help you define yourself, consider that you are a tile in a much larger, colorful mosaic in which each tile is reinforced by the presence of the other.

What Are Your Strengths?

With every person comes a unique set of qualities. Some may call them *strengths* or *weaknesses*, but really they are two sides of the same coin. Some people are very thorough in analysis, thinking through every side of a problem before making a decision. Others respond instinctively to the same situation and make a snap judgment. Which is right? Neither—and both. It simply depends on the organization, its objectives, and the kinds of qualities other people in the organization may have. A CEO who is aware of her own propensity to make quick, instinctive decisions may want a vice president for operations who will be analytical and slow her down a bit to balance her own style. And notice the use of the word *style*. There is nothing wrong or right about either style—it just is what it is. So in this context, when we use the word *strengths* as in "What are your strengths?"—consider it as a question about your skills. In this example, either instinctive or analytical decision-making skills may be considered a singular (and useful) *strength*. Interviewers often ask about *strengths* and *weaknesses*. We will discuss the response to that in more detail later, but it is important here to point out that, most of the time, a strength is merely the flip side of a weakness or vice versa. For example, the "weakness" of the person who is analytical, thorough in considering every conceivable risk to a decision, might reflect an unwillingness to take risks or an unwillingness to come to a meaningful conclusion in a limited period of time with limited information. Likewise, the person who can cut to the quick and make decisions in short order may be impetuous and assume too much risk by being oblivious to it. While neither of these are *right* or *wrong*, the sum of *strengths* and *weaknesses* comprise a leader's *style*. For now, focus on strengths.

How Do You Achieve?

Likewise, knowing how you achieve is important. Do you learn more by reading or listening to others? Do you prefer to work on projects alone, or are you more comfortable working collaboratively with others? Do you like being an advisor or do you like making decisions? Do you like things to be incredibly fast paced with a problem surfacing every few minutes, or do you prefer a slower pace with time to fully consider whatever may be at hand? Do you prefer to be under pressure and busy? Or do you prefer to have some time for "loose ends" and relaxation? Understanding these questions can help you identify work environments best suited to you. Again, none of this is "right" or "wrong," but rather simply a matter of style and preferences about how to work. This can guide you in helping to find an appropriate professional setting where you can make a positive contribution and feel a sense of accomplishment about it.

Likewise, you should consider not only things like pace and team, but you should consider various settings and positions: those interests will vary based on the kind of work that needs to be done and it is as important to consider as well as the setting. For example, you think you need a high-paced setting. You are set and raring to go. There is this great job in physician relations. The community is growing rapidly and the hospital is working hard to grow just as fast, recruiting physicians and keeping them in the hospital's referral network. Somebody needs to keep on top of negotiating agreements with the physicians for office space, loan guarantees, student loan re-payment agreements, contracted employees, management services—whatever it takes to keep the physicians satisfied with your organization (legally), so they keep referring patients to your hospital. But there is just one problem. You are an introvert who likes to work with spreadsheets and data. Yes, you like a fast pace, but with data and calculations. Pretty clearly, this job is not a *fit* for you. Even though the people are terrific and the setting is everything you want, the nature of the work just does not square with your aspirations. We will talk more about "fit" in Chapter 9, but this is a good example of a situation where this is no fit. "How" do you achieve is an important question for you. But "where" you want to achieve it is also an important question for you.

Where Do You Belong?

Consider the results of Exercise 1-1 along with your responses to the previous two questions. Where do *you* think you belong? In thinking about this question, focus on what it is that really excites you. Do you find the lean management structure of a physician practice exciting because you get to do so many different things? Or do you feel overwhelmed at the absence of specialization and prefer to work in a larger organization where the subject-matter span of your activity would be narrower? Are you passionate about sales? Do you find yourself with a passion for children? For the elderly? Where you belong is, in part, where you feel the most reward for performing. It is the "thing" that drives you. Why do you want to get *this* particular degree? What is it about health care that gets your juices flowing? And what part of health care energizes you the most?

DETERMINING YOUR LEGACY

It is doubtful that you have considered much about what kind of legacy you will choose to leave behind after you are gone. And some of this is pretty simple—meaning not complex, but it *is* hard—it will force you to think and also generate some emotion: What do you want out of life and when will you know you have achieved it? By the way, this is about more than mere money—the amalgamation of money is *not* a life objective. (And if that *really* is your mission, you should seriously consider a different career.) Do you want to be the leader of a large academic medical center, or perhaps the executive director of a small nursing home? Does negotiating about money interest you? Then perhaps a managed care organization, or becoming a contract manager in the provider side of the equation, might be for you. Do you like analyzing data, using it to outline a solution to a larger problem? Planning or helping to manage population health might be good fits for you. What you want from life is an outcome of everything we have discussed up to this point; and so is the part about knowing when you have achieved it.

ROUNDING OUT THE ELEMENTS

At this juncture you have done some exercises and reading that, hopefully, have increased your sense of self-awareness. There are two more exercises you should complete to tie all these loose ends together. By now, you should have established a more thorough

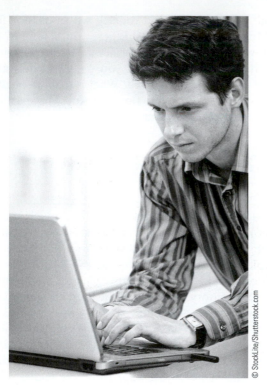

Figure 1-3 What do you want people to say when you are gone?

understanding of your inner self; know more about how you function; and have an idea about where you belong. These are tiles in the mosaic; now you need to put all this good material into one place, one work of art, to help sharpen your focus on your lives and your careers. (See Figure 1-3.)

Management scholar Steven Covey (1989) said, "Begin with the end in mind." Truthfully, this is a common project management technique—you do not just start laying bricks to build a building; you start with what uses you want the building to accommodate and what it should look like. The analogue of this plan, for you, is to write an obituary. Begin with the end in mind; what do you want people to say about you when you are gone; what legacy do you want to leave? Do you want people to mention that you served your community and health organization faithfully for 30 years? Do you want it observed

that you were focused on family first, foremost, and always? Whatever the answers to these questions, these will be your legacy.

Finally, after you have done the previous three exercises, write a one-page memo that best defines why you are in health care. What interests do you aspire to serve now and throughout your life? Use the material from the first three exercises and apply them to this, the fourth exercise.

CONCLUSION

At the end of this chapter, you should be feeling pretty emotionally drained. Good. That means you took this voyage in self-exploration seriously. If you have done that, then you are on your way to defining yourself for the outside world, most notably prospective employers. As we said at the outset, how can you explain yourself to prospective employers if you do not know who you are? Overall, these exercises in the text help answer the question "Who are you?"

If you want to explore this further, you might check out the Human Metrics website. This offers a variety of human behavior measurement devices. Some are free; for some there is a small fee. The Jung Typology Test located at this site is very helpful in understanding a bit more about behavioral characteristics. (See http://www.humanmetrics. com.) A word of caution: These are relatively small tests and may have some limitation in interpreting the results. But as a way of learning more about how to assess self and for a measure of substance in that self-assessment, these kinds of assessments are interesting and helpful. Now that you have a better understanding of self-identity, you can move ahead to the notion of how to put together the best representation of yourself that you can in order to develop a gainful, interesting, and meaningful career (Humanmetrics, 2011).

Another source to consider is the Myers-Briggs Type Indicator®, which provides a 16-cell table of personality types that are useful in balancing traits for building teams, assuring that teams have a mix of people who are both analytical and instinctive; introverted and extraverted, for example (Myers & Briggs Foundation, n.d.) This is based on the work of Carl Jung, so it will be similar to the Jung Typology Test noted above.

Finally, one more source to use to help you identify strengths and weaknesses is *Strength Finders 2.0* (Rath, 2007). If you purchase the book, you can access the online assessment tool that produces a report indicating strong parts of your personality and aspects that you might not find quite as interesting. This is all OK. There is no "right" and "wrong" to any of the outcomes for MBTI or Strengths Finders or any of the other assessment tools—be clear about that. They are only tools that assess characteristics of your personality into certain typologies. They are useful so you—or others such as your supervisors, team leaders, or bosses—can pair you with others who have compensating strengths and who may have weaknesses where you have strengths. Have you heard the saying "There is strength in numbers"? Well, the "numbers" get even stronger if you can balance the people on the team by their various strengths in order to produce a team that has a good balance of talent and ability.

This is why knowing yourself is important. It will help you discover what kind of setting in which you want to work. It will help you discover what kind of work you want to do. It can help you define what it is you want to achieve while you are on this earth. It can also help you discover the kind of people with whom you would be most compatible in the work place. If you can identify all of that within yourself before you even sit down to write the application letter, you are already ahead in the game.

EXERCISES

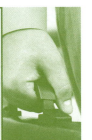

1-1. Take 30 to 60 minutes to write a response to each of the following questions:

- **a.** Where are you from?
- **b.** How does where you are from influence you?
- **c.** What are your values?
- **d.** Who influences you?
- **e.** Who do you admire?
- **f.** What is important to you?

1-2. Take 30 to 60 minutes to write a response to each of the following questions:

- **a.** What are your strengths?
- **b.** How do you achieve? Do you prefer to work alone or as part of a group? Do you prefer to write or speak? Do you prefer to read or listen?
- **c.** Where do you belong?

1-3. Take 30 to 60 minutes to write responses to the following questions:

- **a.** What do you want in life?
- **b.** When will you know you have achieved it? (Money is *not* the objective.)
- **c.** Write a minimum of two paragraphs for each question so you can explain your thinking. Alternative Optional Exercise: Write your own obituary.

1-4. Write a single page, single space, essay responsive to this question: Why do you want a career in health care?

BIBLIOGRAPHY

Bennis, W., & Goldsmith, J. (1997). *Learning to Lead.* Cambridge, MA: Perseus Books.

Bureau of the Census. (1980, n.d.). *Figure 9.* Retrieved April 17, 2012, from Census.gov: http://www2.census.gov/prod2/decennial/documents/1980/1980censusofpopu8011u_bw.pdf

Bureau of the Census. (1980, n.d.). *Table 40.* Retrieved April 17, 2012, from Census. gov: http://www2.census.gov/prod2/decennial/documents/1980/1980censusofpopu80 11u_bw.pdf

Bureau of the Census. (1994, December n.d.). *How We're Changing: Demographic State of the Nation: 1995.* Retrieved April 17, 2012, from Census.gov: http://www.census.gov /prod/1/pop/p23-188.pdf

Bureau of the Census, U.S. (2013). *Quickfacts.* Retrieved February 17, 2014, from Census. gov: http://quickfacts.census.gov/qfd/states/00000.html

Covey, S. R. (1989). *The Seven Habits of Highly Effective People.* New York City: Simon and Schuster.

Drucker, P. (1999). Managing Oneself. *Harvard Business Review*, 64–75.

Dye, C. F. (2000). *Leadership in Healthcare.* Chicago: Health Administration Press.

Goleman, D. (1995). *Emotional Intelligence.* New York City: Bantam Books.

Holmes, O. W. (n.d.). *BrainyQuote.com.* Retrieved October 3, 2013, from http://www .brainyquote.com/

Humanmetrics. (2011, n.d.). *Jung Typology Test.* Retrieved April 8, 2012, from Human Metrics: http://www.humanmetrics.com/cgi-win/jtypes2.asp

Myers & Briggs Foundation. (n.d.). *The MBTI Instrument for Live.* Retrieved October 3, 2013, from myersbriggs.org: http://www.myersbriggs.org/

Rath, T. (2007). *Strengths Finder 2.0.* New York City: Gallup Press.

Seidman, D. (2007). *How: Why HOW We Do Anything Means Everything.* Hoboken, NJ: John Wiley & Sons.

Starr, P. (1982). *The Social Transformation of American Medicine.* New York: Harper Collins/ Basic Books.

Chapter 2

You Never Get a Second Chance to Make a First Impression

Call it corny or trite or overused, but it is as true as it is simple: there *is* only one "first impression." Everyone you meet—everyone—is a potential:

- Employer
- Reference
- Mentor/advisor
- Friend
- Network contact
- LinkedIn contact
- Facebook friend

So what does this mean to you? It means that you should always dress appropriately for the context; be professional; uphold your end of the bargain in group work for classes; be on time for meetings (and classes!); and participate in groups, meetings (and classes!) in affirmative ways.

THE LOOK

When a guest speaker visits your class or your professional club, dress for the occasion. If it is a class, you should be in professional attire. There are some good examples in the photographs on this page and the next. Take a look at the guy in Figure 2-1; there are a couple of things to note. First, to have a professional look, it does *not* need to be a black or dark suit, though you can never really go wrong with a

dark suit. This gray looks terrific on this young man. Also note the shirt is a very nice contrast to the gray. Also notice that he has just a little bit—¼ to ½ of an inch—of shirt sleeve showing at the cuff. Finally, look at that knot in the tie—perfectly tied. This is a detailed "together" look. This says this young man is on top of his game; you can put some faith in what he says because he has "the look" that says "I pay attention to detail and to my surroundings; and I have respect for you and what you do." Likewise, see the young woman in Figure 2-2. This is a

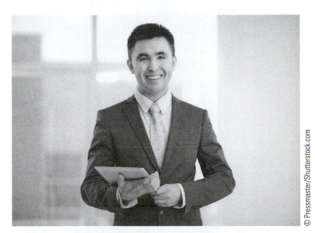

© Pressmaster/Shutterstock.com

Figure 2-1 An example of a professional outfit for a male.

dark suit; the coloring fits the complexion of the woman wearing it; note that the blouse is a subtle but clear contrast to the suit. This is a "quiet, conservative" look. The skirt ends slightly above the knee, and you see a similar look in Figure 2-3 with a pants suit—also very appropriate.

Color of suit is important. While it is not typical for men to wear bright colored suits, it is certainly appropriate for women on some occasions. The interview or professional networking event is *not* one of them. Likewise, the men should avoid attention-grabbing styles or colors. You do not want to look like a member of the latest boy band; you are going for the executive look here.

I should add a word about "skirt" or "slacks" (pants suit). First, let us be clear a "pants suit" is just that. It is a jacket and slacks that are uniform in material and styled to go together. Wearing a jacket and slacks is not a suit—for either men or women. Second, either one—pant or skirt—is

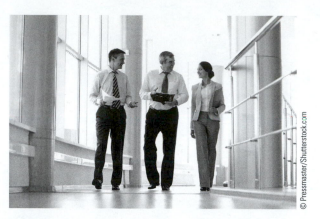

Figure 2-3 Female professional wearing a pants suit.

appropriate, but just make certain the skirt is an appropriate length. The mini-skirt that rises four inches above your knee does *not* suggest a focus on professionalism. The other fashion issue for women is the matter of cleavage. Showing too much—which in the business context really means *any*—is not going to help you. Whether the interviewer is male or female, you will be penalized for too much décolletage. They will be embarrassed, as well. Figure 2-2 represents a look that hits the right tone.

Both Figures 2-1 and 2-2 represent the "business professional" look. This is the right kind of look for the interview to be certain; it is also the look for a national convention of a professional association or the local chapter meeting; the guest lecturer in class; or the networking event hosted by your student club. Why? Because every one of the people you will meet at these events is a potential employer, reference, mentor and advisor. You want to look professional. You want to look this way because of what it says to them about you: As discussed above, that you are "on your game," that you pay attention to detail, that you respect them and what they do. If you do not believe this, go to class when you have a guest speaker and dress in jeans you have not washed since last semester and a T-shirt. Look around. How do you feel? How do you *think* this looks to the guest speaker? (I do not recommend actually *doing* this; just imagine it.)

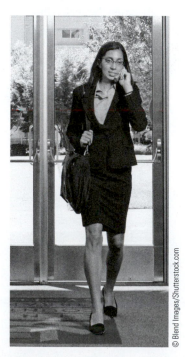

Figure 2-2 An example of a professional outfit for a female.

Business casual is something that can be a bit tricky. Business casual means attire that would be appropriate for business, but that is not the "full dress uniform." Both Figures 2-4 and 2-5 are good examples. Note the crisp look that works for business but is not quite as detailed or "finished" as full business professional. This look is also good for the networking event hosted by your student club. It is also a good look for some professional conventions or local meetings. The key here is to know the culture of the organization before deciding "business professional" or "business casual."

Casual is not the same as "business casual." Figures 2-6 and 2-7 are good examples of "casual." Note there are no ties or ascots or scarves in the examples. The sweater is a good accessory, except in

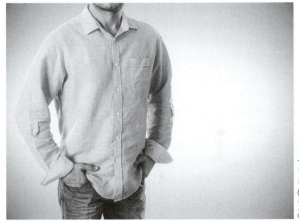

Figure 2-6 Casual outfit for a male.

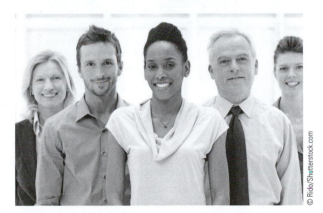

Figure 2-4 Examples of business casual outfits.

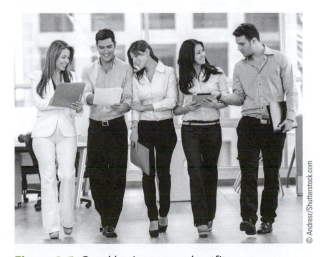

Figure 2-5 Co-ed business casual outfits.

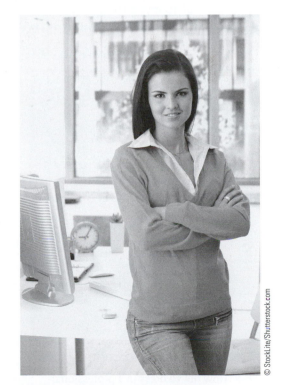

Figure 2-7 Casual outfit for a female.

warm climates. The guy in Figure 2-6 has his shirt out, which is the appropriate way to wear a casual shirt. This is the *only* time a gentleman's shirt should not be tucked. For women, again, casual can be either slacks or skirt. Crop pants are a nice look; the skirt can be shorter for this occasion, but remember, you are still among fellow professionals. What impression do you want to create in *their* eyes?

Figures 2-8 and 2-9 are here as examples of what *not* to do—at least not outside the privacy of your own home. At this point you are thinking, "yeah but he does not mean class." Yes, I do. Dress casual to class, but nothing less. Why? Remember what I said about *everyone* you meet being a potential employer, reference, mentor, etc. Every faculty member you meet is a potential reference. Even if members of the faculty do not always do the "full dress uniform," they do notice *your* appearance. You will need them as a reference. So in addition to doing the work in class, you should present an appearance that says you want to enter the profession. "Grad student" and "undergrad grunge" hardly suggest the

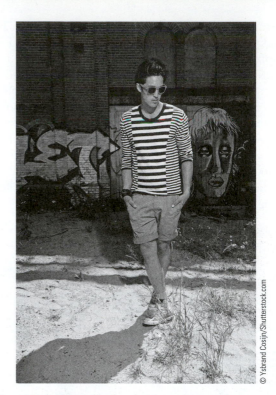

Figure 2-9 Example of an inappropriate outfit.

image of a budding young professional, so do not dress like that. For a bit more detail on the "interview fashion" scene, see the box called "Sidebar on Fashion."

THE SOUND

Consider this scenario: you are going to the class with the guest lecturer or the professional convention networking event. You have gone to a lot of trouble—the right suit, excellent shirt or blouse, perfectly tied tie and coifed hair. You look terrific. You walk into the event. Confident. Ready. Your chance to talk to "THE star" of the event or a "bigwig VP" arises. You walk up, extend your hand for the great handshake (see the sidebar on the etiquette of the handshake), and you say: "Hey, Sam, great speech. Does your hospital take interns, because I need one this summer to graduate."

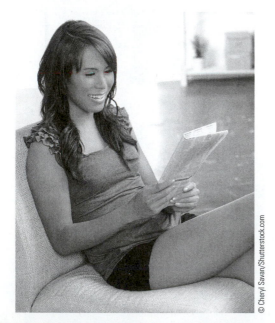

Figure 2-8 How not to dress in a professional environment.

SIDEBAR ON FASHION

It is way beyond the scope of this book to talk much about fashion, but there are some basics. If you want to follow up on this, do a bit of research—there are some very good books and sources regarding color, patterns, tones, and how to bring them all together. The material here is more basic. As a general observation that applies to both genders, it is always better to be too "conservative" in dress than too "liberal." You will be better off if the "first impression" is one that says, "This person is pretty reserved" than one that says, "Way too casual for this organization." It is easier, in this respect, to move from a more "conservative" style to a more "casual" style than the other way around. In addition, it is important to add a note here about tattoos and body piercings. Keep the tattoos hidden. Keep the body piercings conservative if you must have them. For young men, it is still controversial, in health care, to have an earpiece. For young women, pierced ears have been around forever—just wear conservative earrings and not some dangly thing that distracts from your overall appearance. Things like nose rings and tongue and lip "barbells" should disappear. These are inappropriate in health care in any setting. There are health risks with tongue piercings in particular. In any event, this type of body art is not mainstream and will merely be a negative distraction in an interview (or any other professional) setting.

For gentlemen: If you have gone to the trouble and expense of getting a great looking suit, be certain the shirt is appropriate. If you have a 34-inch sleeve, but borrowed a dress shirt from the guy who played center on your high school basketball team, it probably is not going to fit correctly. Make sure the shirt sleeves extend beyond the suit sleeves about ½ inch but no more than a full inch. Likewise, do not wear a loud color shirt or one with big patterns. Stick with a solid white or light blue with a pinpoint collar. As for the tie, make certain it blends or contrasts "quietly" with the suit. If you are in a dark gray suit, you have some flexibility here and can use a splash of color to complete

the look. Stay with a diagonal pattern of stripes or pattern that complements the suit. Pay attention to all the detail—from head to toe, including shoes and socks. Make sure the socks are appropriate to the suit and the shoes. If you are wearing a dark blue suit, you should have dark blue or black socks. Your shoes should be black, brown, or cordovan (and the belt should be the same color as the shoes), depending on the suit, most likely black or brown. With a suit, laced shoes are always appropriate, though dressy loafers are also acceptable. Regardless of color, make sure they are clean and shined and do not look like they have been run over by a bus and then dragged from a car. The last item here to discuss is the length of your pants. Again, the wrong length here can really harm all the good work you have done so far to look good. The pant length should be such that the front crease "breaks" at the top of your foot. In other words, the pants should meet the top of the shoe and, in effect, rest on it to the point where there is a slight dimple in the crease of the slacks. Pants that stop at your ankle, or pants that reach under the heel of your shoe, are both wrong and destroy the look you are trying to achieve.

For women: As I mentioned earlier, either a skirt or pant suit is acceptable. For pants, the same basic rule regarding length applies: There should be a slight dimple or "break" in the crease just above the top of the shoe. As to skirts, anything shorter than just above the knee may cast an unprofessional look. For hosiery, it depends on season and geography. Bare legs are much more the custom in the southern part of the United States for the very practical reason that the temperature is hotter there for much more of the year than in the north. If you show up for an interview in January in Minneapolis with bare legs someone might question your judgment. Be mindful of season and geography—and organizational culture if you have a sense of it. As for shoes, the four-inch platform heel, or the six-inch spike heel, is not the look you want.

(continues)

(continued)

Many professional women wear shorter heels—2 to 3 inches perhaps. In the case of a hospital setting, be sure they are practical and closed toe. Regardless of all else, make sure you can walk comfortably in them. The color of the shoe is more seasonable for women than men. Black is always acceptable; however, at different times of the year or in different parts of the country, a camel or neutral tone could be appropriate. As to the suit or dress you wear to the interview, be conservative. Women have a bit more flexibility in this respect than men because there are so many colors and patterns available in women's clothing. As a general proposition, having gone to the trouble to make sure the skirt length and shoe heel is correct, you might want to reconsider the fire-engine red dress adorned with sequins. Avoid loud colors and overly bright pastels for both suits and blouses. Women have more options regarding accessories than men, but the same basic rule applies. Avoid loud colors and weird patterns; stay with complimentary colors between the blouse, suit, and scarf if you use one.

For both: Make sure your choice of suit or dress is well pressed and dry-cleaned prior to the interview. Likewise, the shirt or blouse should be either laundered or dry-cleaned and pressed. You have gone to a lot of trouble to "dress for success," so do not let some wrinkles get in the way. A lot of dry cleaners also do alterations, so that skirt or those pants can be corrected, if necessary. Also, if you purchase a suit for an interview, then the typical full service retail store should provide alterations at no cost. Speaking of purchasing a suit, etc., if you live near an outlet mall, then I strongly suggest hunting there for that perfect suit, dress, tie, shirt, and accessory. This is a lot less costly than paying full retail, though you will most likely need to go elsewhere for the alterations.

If you travel for an interview and, despite your best efforts to pack so things will not wrinkle, your shirt or suit comes out of the suitcase looking like you have slept in them for the last four nights, all is not lost. Hotels have irons and ironing boards. Or you can try the low-labor fix of hanging the affected item(s) in the bathroom and turn on the shower to a scalding hot temperature, leave the room and close the door. Let the water run 20 to 30 minutes. Then retrieve the suit or shirt, hang it up, and give it about one hour to absorb the steam. This will resolve most small wrinkles. Of course, it is not at all environmentally friendly because of the wasted water, but it does work. The best solution is to iron the piece(s) if you can do it without (a) burning the item and (b) starting a three-alarm fire.

SIDEBAR FOR HANDSHAKE

Members of the human race have been shaking hands for thousands of years. While some cultures use a different form of greeting—a slight bow, for example in Japan—the western custom is to greet someone with a handshake. But if you have done a lot of this, you know there are some "wet fish" and some "bone crushers." There are some people who use this as occasion to pull you toward them. Those traits all say something about them: The "wet fish" may likely be a person with little self-confidence; the other two may be controlling personalities. So with this in mind, you want to present yourself as confident and willing to serve.

As you introduce yourself, extend your right arm at about waist level. Your palm can be vertical to the floor; tilted upward slightly; turned completely up; or turned completely down. Each of these is a commentary on you. I recommend you keep your palm slightly tilted up. This says you are open, genuine. A full palm up is a bit submissive. A full palm down could be a controlling, "I am superior" personality. As your hand meets the other person's hand, make sure the web of

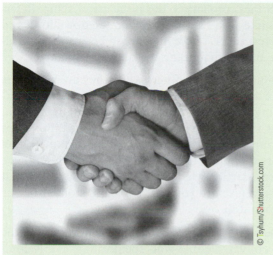

Figure 2-10 The *web to web* basic business handshake.

your hand—that space between your thumb and index finger—meets the other person's web. Use a firm grip. Again, you do not want to make the blood in their hand rush to their head. And you do not want someone asking themself, "Can't this person engage?" Greet the other person with a nice, firm grip. Figure 2-10 is a good example of a "web to web" handshake.

Shake—from the elbow—the hand two or three times in no more than three or four seconds. If it lasts more than that, the other person will become uncomfortable. If you shake from the shoulder, you will just be jolting the other person—same result: uncomfortable.

If you are a gentleman, when meeting a woman wait for her to extend her hand. If she does so, then engage in the handshake as described above. If not, then a nod and polite smile will suffice. In addition, particularly for the men, there is a subconscious phenomenon that occurs sometimes. There is a

predisposition for men to address women by their first name, while addressing men with the traditional "Mr." title. Likewise, too many male students refer to male faculty members as "Dr." while calling a woman faculty member (who also has a PhD) "Mrs." This is entirely inappropriate. In the case of MDs or PhDs, it is *always* "doctor" regardless of gender. Otherwise, it is "Ms." as much as it is "Mr." To do otherwise is disrespectful.

Use just your right hand. The "two hand grip," in a business setting, is inappropriately forward. If the other person is someone with whom you have had a long standing relationship and know well, then go ahead. But generally, the two hand grip is seen as artificially friendly, especially when used the first time you meet someone. It has been called the "politician's grip." Another form of informality that is somewhat less obtrusive is to use your left hand to touch the other person's right elbow. This, too, suggests familiarity, friendship, and openness, and probably is inappropriate for a first meeting.

If you have just washed your hands, make certain they are dry before engaging with a handshake. Likewise, if your hands are full—or if the other person's hands are full—a simple nod and smile will be sufficient. Sometimes people may have sweaty hands; if you shake hands with such a person, do *not* immediately wipe your hand on your pants or skirt. Do not reach for the hand sanitizer dispenser. That will just embarrass them further. Clean your hand later in discretion.

Make eye contact during the time of this greeting. It says you are confident and forthright: two things you want prospective employers and colleagues to think of you.

Finally, avoid "the fives" (low, medium, or high) and fist bumps unless you are with your own peer group. People who make hiring decisions probably are sufficiently older and they may not "get it."

This is an approach guaranteed to get you attention that will not help. First, it is grammatically incorrect. (*Hint: Do you need an "intern" or an "internship"?*) Second, the speaker or guest is very likely 10 to 15 or more years older than you—use of the first name

is *only* appropriate if you know the person *and* they have said the use of their first name is OK, or they are a family friend. Beyond that, how sincere does "great speech" sound in the context of what this guy is saying? Do you suppose the guest speaker *really* thinks he did a good job and got through to this guy, or is he thinking "What a flake?" Additionally, asking about internship in this way seems both awkward and phony. It makes much more sense to establish a rapport with the speaker before jumping into the internship requirements. Oh, by the way, it is *not* just about what *you* need. The key ingredient in any of these conversations with potential employers or internship preceptors is the notion of how you can add value to the organization. What can you do for them? You will read more about this matter further along in the book, but you might as well start thinking about it sooner rather than later.

It is critically important to reflect your professionalism in the way you speak. "Mr. Jones, thank you for taking the time to speak to our class today. I enjoyed your remarks. Do you have a business card? I would like to have an opportunity to visit with you, but do not want to interfere with your meeting my classmates." *This* tells the listener that you: (a) are considerate of him and others—you do not monopolize his time in a crowd; (b) understand the custom of exchanging business cards; and (c) want more of his time. This all demonstrates self-awareness, confidence, and seriousness. The *good* executives will *find* the time to talk with you. There is a talent shortage out there. Be the person who is going to fill that gap—in appearance, in voice, and beyond.

A Review of Some Basics

When you speak, do not drop the "g" from "ing." Avoid vernacular like "hangin' around." Here is where you need to move from backpack to briefcase; use of the language is important to establishing yourself as a professional.

Related to "hangin' around" is the garbled voice—or mumbling. Enunciate what you intend to say clearly. Make it easy for others to hear and understand. When you do not fully pronounce words, or talk with your mouth mostly closed—or worse while you have something in it—it strains the listener's ear. If you want to move up, if you want to be considered professional, look, and *sound* the part.

Another corollary to this is the use of slang. References like "411" and "keepin' on the down low" and "I'm just sayin' " have no place in business conversations. Be stylish in using the language suitably.

Do not interrupt others while they are speaking. There are few more disrespectful things than interrupting others. It says "I am not listening to you. What I have to say is more important." Be aware of yourself in these settings and be certain you let others complete their thought and their sentence before asserting whatever it is you intend to say that has been given to you as if carved in stone from the mountaintop.

Use appropriate volume. The listener is not in the next county. People who speak in an overly loud voice seem to be compensating for an insecurity of some kind: They *really need* to be heard. Likewise, however, do not speak so softly that you are hard to hear. People might think you are uncertain about what you are saying. Or, perhaps worse, they might mishear what you actually said. Make it easy for the listener to—well, listen to you. Part of that is clarity of voice, etc. When speaking with others, be sure to speak at an appropriate volume. Be conversational; project but do not be overbearing about it. Be confident and express what you have to say in a normal tone of voice; you can use volume and pace of speech to emphasize various points along the way.

Be respectful and slightly formal. Our culture has changed quite a bit in the way we treat each other, particularly when it comes to "rank." People who have been out of school and in the profession for a good long time may not understand when a graduating senior looking for a job calls them by their first name; especially, if they are meeting for the first time. You may think you are equals; perhaps your future boss does as well, but what if that person is 55 years old, COO of the hospital and, let us just say, a little "old school." You walk in looking like a million bucks, extend your hand and say, "Hi, Jack." To him this will seem like fingernails on a chalk board—pretty presumptuous, while it may be "normal" for you. It is pretty likely that in the job search process you will meet people who are your elders. When you do, use their proper title and last name, as in, "It is a pleasure to meet you, Mr./Ms./Dr. Smith." In addition, at least initially, use "sir" or "ma'am" as appropriate. As in this exchange:

Mr. Smith: Welcome to our hospital, Ms. Jones, please have a seat.
Ms. Jones: Thank you, sir.

A "Yes, sir" or "No ma'am" used intermittently throughout the conversation will go a long way toward making the point that you are respectful, serious, interested in them, and know how to behave appropriately. You need to sort of "feel" your way with this. It does not need to be used with each and every question and answer. That can seem obsequious. If you want to emphasize a point, it is a good appendage to the answer. All of this can also apply to people who may be only five years older than you. Even if they are relatively young and still hip, they may prefer for you to recognize their status by being a bit deferential in this respect. A simple rule to follow: unless someone says "Call me by my first name"—do not.

Finally, and this certainly is *not* the least important, look people in the eye when you are speaking or listening to them. This does not mean a staring contest to see who "breaks" first; it is, however, to say that if you do not look the interviewer in the eye, you will be seen as less than completely candid. Who wants to be considered disingenuous in a job interview? You should "break" eye contact from time to time, but your overall attention should be on the person with whom you are having the conversation. Otherwise, you are wasting your time and theirs.

In summary, your interview or meeting should be with a clear voice, at an appropriate volume, free of vernacular and slang, and clearly spoken. Be aware of your surroundings; do not interrupt others when they are speaking; be courteous and polite. And, of course, nothing can replace solid preparation. All of this is, in a sense, "packaging." So, if you have done the appropriate homework in advance, do not waste that effort. Put it in the right spoken context. There will be more about interviews in Chapters 6 and 7.

THE WRITTEN WORD

This section is about basic writing. Because the cover letter is critically important, it will be treated separately in Chapter 5. The next several pages, however, are dedicated to the number one issue among employers. Ask any executive what the biggest concern they have about young professionals joining their organization, and one of the top answers is sure to be "They cannot write." Somewhere along the way in education, teaching the skill of writing became a secondary concern. I am not talking about writing in the sense of being able to phrase alluring alliteration or engaging in pithy phrases of pinpoint facts; this is about the ability to write a complete sentence correctly punctuated. In addition, appropriate use of verbs, nouns, and pronouns is more important than some apparently believe.

Follow basic grammar rules. If you are not sure about the difference between a comma and a semicolon or a noun and a pronoun, or a verb and an adverb, find out and use them appropriately. To refresh your skills and knowledge about writing, get a copy of *Grammar and Writing Skills for the Health Professional* (Villemaire, 2007). It is intended as a refresher for things like nouns, pronouns, verbs; how to organize for writing; and how to construct a paragraph. It is a complete "how to" in a pretty concise package. For the quick look-up to a specific question, check out http://owl.english.purdue.edu (Purdue University, 1995). This is a dynamite website that provides a terrific review of proper use of the English language. For a comedic way of thinking about punctuation in depth, see a small book called *Eats, Shoots and Leaves*, by Lynne Truss. The apocryphal story is about the panda that enters a café. He orders a sandwich, eats it, then draws a gun and fires two shots into the air and leaves. As the panda was making his way out the door, the waiter asked why he would engage in such odd behavior. The panda replied, "I'm a panda; look it up." The waiter did and he found the definition of panda: "Large black-and-white bear-like mammal, native to China. Eats, shoots and leaves." All of this for the lowly—and misplaced—comma after "eats" (Truss, 2003).

Spelling

Do not simply rely on the spell-check that comes with your word processing program. Consider that the *beginning* of your spelling and typographical error-checking process. Often times the spell-check on your computer will let pass correctly spelled words that are used in the wrong context. Whenever you write something, do it far enough in advance that you can set it aside for—best case two or three days; worst case a couple of hours—so you can reread it with a fresh eye. (By the way, *ours* is one of those words that would be OK with the spell-check if I had somehow written it here without the *h*.)

Sentences

Be mindful of sentence structure. A sentence should express a complete thought. It can be simple, or it can be complex, but in any event, it should not run on to embrace more than one concept, nor should it fall short of putting a noun and verb together in a way that finishes the thought. Now, *that* sentence was pretty long, but not a run on. A run-on sentence is one with too many concepts, nouns, and verbs that do not belong together. A fragmented sentence is one that does not finish what it starts. Usually, a noun or verb is left hanging without a partner.

Spacing and Margins

Adopt a style. The style you adopt may be one of several, as there are several correct ways to do this. Use a ragged right margin, or not, but be consistent. Indent at the beginning of a new paragraph. If you, in a single-spaced document, put an extra line between the paragraphs, then do not indent. For memos and letters alike, some like to have justified right and left margins, single spaced, with an extra line between paragraphs. Others prefer single spaced, ragged right margin and indent for each new paragraph with no extra line between them. Others prefer double spaced. Usually, in this case, one indents the new paragraph without the extra line between them as four lines between two paragraphs would look strange. Perhaps the two most important points here are to adopt a style that is easy to read and be consistent with its use. The other important point here is to

be cognizant of what the organization for which you are working may require. Oftentimes, organizations will have a form of stylebook or a set of preferences for how memos should be structured (particularly as to heading, etc.) that will dictate this to you. Follow *that* style as opposed to using your own.

People and Objects

What is wrong with the following sentence? "I know many people that want to avoid going to the hospital."

With the use of *that* in referring to *people* those people just became inanimate objects—and they are not—they are *people*. When referring to *people*—and this includes any label that we might attach to people like *patients*, *physicians*, *administrators*, and the like, use *who* (or in some cases *whom*, but that is beyond the scope of this book). The use of *that* is for inanimate or nonhuman objects only. For example, "We have a needs assessment program that helps match our patient needs with our services" and "We have a needs assessment coordinator who is outstanding at her job."

THE ABUSE—AND POSITIVE USE—OF SOCIAL MEDIA

Surely you have heard by now that you need to be a bit circumspect about what you post on your favorite social media sites. Employers are now routinely searching social media for entries posted by prospective employees. This material can say a *lot* about the kind of person you are. Is what you have on your Facebook page consistent with the person you described in Chapter 1? If you regard yourself as a values-centered person, why have photos of yourself downing beer through a funnel, or pictures of yourself so revealing that they damage your professional image. In fact, these are the very things that will disqualify you with employers. Forty-five percent of employers now research social media backgrounds of potential employees and 35% of those found reasons not to hire candidates based on what they saw on the applicant's social page website (Grove, 2009).

The same study, conducted by Harris Interactive for CareerBuilders.com, found that provocative photos, sharing of drugs and alcohol, and bad-mouthing former employers were top reasons for not selecting candidates. Posting comments and pictures about vacations, family gatherings, events, and so forth are fine so long as they do not portray you as an overindulgent, postadolescent party animal. First, just avoid that behavior—it is fraught with its own risks. Second, if you do have a "night out," think twice before posting photos of it for the entire world to see.

The other danger in this genre is getting tagged looking like an idiot in somebody else's social media page. Assuming this person is a friend, you need to approach them to get it cleaned up. Indeed, they are most likely near the same age as you, so should be doing this for themselves as they look for *their* internship or job. Put it to them that way: This is in their own best interest. And if they resist, you can at least ask them to do you the favor of taking down photos with your face in them. You do not need to be dragged down by someone else's poor judgment.

While there are legal issues about employers using this material as grounds to reject prospective employees, there is no doubt this is going to continue happening. So, until the legal questions are resolved, expect employers to be aggressive about using social media to screen applicants. Among the things employers have found are the following: T-shirts with racist remarks; driving while holding a beer; drug use; bad-mouthing former employers; and lying about qualifications (Johnson, 2012).

Using Social Media to Your Advantage

The social media outlets need not be something from which you run or contain material you want to hide. I have discussed avoiding the "negative" material above. But Facebook, LinkedIn, Twitter, and the rest can be your tool in building a "brand" of yourself so your prospective employer can learn more of your strengths, skills, and character; they can also be your tool for marketing to help employers discover you. Think of this as a sort of electronic résumé you can share with everyone with whom you exchange an e-mail. Use social media to your advantage and to cast yourself in a light most favorable to you. This is *not* to say that you should use your creative genius to invent something about yourself that is untrue! Rather, you can depict your strengths.

You went through some self-discovery exercises in Chapter 1. Social media can give you an opportunity to present those values in words and graphics that can come to be your brand, which is a form of marketing yourself. Think of this as taking that person you defined in Chapter 1 and using every avenue available to present that person. Your brand is also represented by your business card, your letterhead (and letter!), your resume, and yes, your wardrobe, but the way to make the broadest impression is through social media.

Have you done something special that was particularly rewarding, like volunteering at the local children's hospital? Get a picture of yourself with a patient (*after* getting written permission from the patient or their parent). You could also post this on Facebook. Use the *Experience* section of LinkedIn to mention your volunteer work. Or, if you have completed a special project that has some graphics or spreadsheets, compile them as a portfolio and put those on Facebook as .jpeg files or mention them in *Experience* in LinkedIn. This will set you apart from others—showing your willingness to give to others; to go the extra mile.

If you have a good professional profile, on LinkedIn, for example, you might consider putting the link in your signature block at the bottom of your e-mail. While this is not for everyone, if you have a knack for digital photography, you might consider doing a YouTube video. You might also consider creating a portfolio of your work, if you do not already have one, and put it on a CD or DVD. Be sure to pay very close attention to detail if you do either of these, and have them reviewed by friends and faculty to make sure they are going to accomplish what you want to accomplish (Schawbel, 2009).

CONCLUSION

A pretty complete list of ways you can connect with everyone around you was provided at the beginning of the chapter. This specifically includes your colleagues in the program. How do you relate to them? If you disagree about something are you willing to discuss it and try to find an accommodation or do you storm out of the room? If they do something that you find annoying do you tolerate it or avoid them? Or mention it to them in some way? When working on group projects, do you uphold your end of the bargain? Do you meet deadlines and have your work available for others to review?

A first-year student (alias *Roy*) once asked a second year student (alias *Cathy*) where she had interned the prior summer. Cathy told him and thought little of it. It was a 10-second exchange, if that. Later that week Cathy received an e-mail from her preceptor. Could she tell the preceptor a little bit about Roy? It seems Roy had e-mailed the preceptor, told the preceptor that Cathy had such a marvelous experience and that Cathy highly recommended that he try to get that internship; he made it sound as if he and Cathy were friends. In fact, of course, Cathy had done no such thing, and she barely knew the guy. Can you imagine her reaction? What does this say about *his* sense of ethical behavior? We learned later he had done basically the same thing with two other people.

The moral of this story is that everyone around you is a potential reference, or employer, or the like. It is also central to the idea that professionalism is not just a suit and a terrific résumé; it is about behavior. Roy proved he still has a lot of learning to do about what it takes. If you think he only burned bridges with three people, guess again. How many times did the three "victims" tell friends and fellow students? Faculty? Roy will not be getting much help from his classmates anytime soon. That is a memory they will carry with them for a long, long time.

In the end, you need to behave ethically to be a true professional. Otherwise, you are merely imitating. See Chapter 9 for a full discussion on ethical behavior. The appearance certainly counts—a proper professional appearance will open some doors, just as the behavior described above will close them. So how you relate to your colleagues in the program is critically important, whether it is as egregious as trying to get an inside track for an internship, or as simple as not being fully engaged as a team player in the group project. This is the beginning of your professional network. Respect and value the people around you and let them see that in your behavior. To the point of this chapter: It will be easier for them to believe that you are serious about the profession and respectful of others if you dress the part appropriately, if you speak properly, and if you write correctly.

Observations from the Professionals

Electronic Networking

Sarah Boyd is the owner of SJBusiness Partners, LLC, a consulting company specializing in service excellence and business development. The firm works with organizations in all industries to positively impact corporate culture, the customer experience, and the bottom line.

Electronic marketing is all about communicating your personal brand story. It is up to you to showcase what makes you unique, your strengths, and your passion, in a professional yet engaging way. Social media can help you do this beautifully or seal your fate.

As health administration students, you have numerous opportunities to connect with professionals who can help you land your first job, serve as a mentor, or introduce you to high-level administrators. It is up to you to take advantage of this opportunity and continue your interaction beyond short in-person encounters. You have already learned about what content should not be on your personal Facebook or Twitter accounts, so I will focus on the use of more "professional" social media platforms here, LinkedIn and Google+.

LinkedIn is a simple way to share your résumé and specific project experience in an environment that is friendly to networking. You must display your own career or internship experience on your profile in a way that is descriptive and yet concise. Here are a few great examples taken from a real health administration student's page:

- Evaluated the current Information Technology (IT) project prioritization process and software for effectiveness and efficiency
- Interviewed IT and executive level IT prioritization stakeholders for a multidisciplinary perspective on the current system
- Created a Gantt timeline and multiple meeting agendas to track project progress
- Presented recommendations through a formal report and presentation to the executive committee where two of four recommendations were immediately implemented

This is also a great place to have recommendations from administrators, professors, or managers. You can request recommendations through LinkedIn and link specific comments with each position held or project completed. These recommendations can be powerful and convey more about you and your character than would be appropriate for you to attempt to communicate. Professors can even give you a recommendation. Here is an example of a recommendation a professor gave a student on LinkedIn that I think is a great example:

"(name of student) appears to possess all the traits needed to be successful as a high-level manager. She is very intelligent and insightful, has great organizational instincts, is a creative thinker, and has a terrific personality."

When connecting with speakers or professionals, make sure to personalize the "Invitation to connect." Remind them where and when you met and say something like "I would love to stay in touch and possibly work together in the future." Too many people use the generic invitation message, and this small step will help you stand out. Join groups that are of interest (i.e., ACHE, MGMA, MHA Alumni Group, etc.) so that you can meet others and participate in the discussion.

Google+ is a good stage for sharing papers you have written, projects you have worked on, or relevant industry articles. Although Google+ is still relatively uncharted territory for most, this portal allows you to store and distribute your work in a way that is easy to access. This profile can combine the perks of a conventional blog and a professional portfolio. Create "circles" within your contact list to allow each post to be personalized to the audience you desire. For example, you could have circles for classmates, alumni, professors, administrators, and other business contacts. Each time you upload a document, you can choose who sees this work. Keep in mind that you will also need to add documents to your "public" circle so that anyone searching for you can see content that will serve as an overview to your interests and background. Google+ also has video conferencing capabilities that can be helpful when working on group projects or as an alternative to a phone call in appropriate situations.

As health administration students, you will need to learn to balance your professional and personal lives in a mature manner. If this balance is not achieved, social media will communicate this message to potential employers and you will pay the price. You will reap the benefits, however, if you make a deliberate effort to establish your personal brand and use social media platforms to communicate your message. Remember to think about content in terms of your audience and be persistent in your efforts. As the journey from health administration students to professional unfolds, be positive and proactive and the cards will fall as they should.

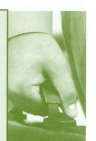

EXERCISES

2-1. Find a fellow student and do a "role play." Practice the "meet the guest speaker" scenario described at pages 14, 17 and 18. One of you is the aspiring student speaking to the guest speaker after their speech. Practice the handshake. Practice introducing yourself. Pay attention to how you speak. I will cover more about "the elevator speech" in Chapter 4—for now, just mention a few things about your educational program. The guest speaker should critique the "student's" performance. Then change roles and do it again.

2-2. Get a partner and review each other's social media spaces. Look for inappropriate behavior, photos, references, and language. Be very detailed! Critique and share the results with your partner. Now do the reverse; look for positive entries in each other's spaces. Critique and share the results.

2-3. Have a colleague review your "Why I want to be in health care" essay. Do the same for them. Look for errors in grammar and punctuation. Are there verbs that are plural and nouns that are singular? Or vice versa? Are the sentences complete? Do the paragraphs form a cohesive thought? Again, pay close attention to detail. Share the results with one another. Use this tool to discover how much general writing help you might need.

2-4. On an occasion where you are required to "dress up," identify the person sitting next to you and review one another's attire. Is the tie well tied and snug against the collar? Is the skirt too short or the top too revealing? Does the suit fit appropriately? Are the colors appropriate? Share this with each other.

BIIBLIOGRAPHY

Grove, J. V. (2009, August 19). *45% of Employers Now Screen Social Media Profiles*. Retrieved March 23, 2012, from Mashable Business: http://mashable.com/2009/08/19 /social-media-screening/

Johnson, S. (2012, February 13). Facebook posts may cost you a job. *The (Charleston, SC) Post and Courier*, pp. 12-D.

Purdue University. (1995). *OWL: Purdue Online Writing Lab*. Retrieved February 5, 2012, from Purdue University website: http://owl.english.purdue.edu/owl/section/1/

Schawbel, D. (2009, January 5). *7 Secrets to Getting Your Next Job Using Social Media*. Retrieved March 13, 2012, from Mashable Business: http://mashable.com/2009/01/05 /job-search-secrets/

Schawbel, D. (2009, February 5). *Branding 101: How to Discover and Create Your Own Brand*. Retrieved March 12, 2012, from Mashable Business: http://mashable .com/2009/02/05/personal-branding-101/

Truss, L. (2003). *Eats, Shoots and Leaves*. New York: Gotham Books.

Villemaire, D. A. (2007). *Grammar and Writing Skills for the Healthcare Professional, 2d Edition*. Clifton Park, NY: Cengage Learning.

Chapter 3

Finding the Right Place: It Is a Big World Out There

Health care is *big* business. Health care-related expenditures represent more than 17% of the gross domestic product (CMSa, 2012). While many think of the obvious venues—hospitals, physician practices, and long-term care facilities—when talking about health care, it is much, much more diverse. The fragmentation in the U.S. health system is frequently discussed, but not often considered when thinking about career opportunities. Some examples of both the size of the industry as well as its fragmentation: 4,500 biotech companies, 6,000 device manufacturers, 5,800 hospitals, and 1,300 health plans (Keckley & Bigalke, 2011). Because delivering medical services is so complex, it has subdivided into a host of categories. Thus, in addition to those mentioned above, consider the following:

- Pharmaceutical companies
- Dietary supplements industry
- Personal care product (medication) industry
- Waste management equipment and plants industry
- Hospital and physician furniture industry
- Medical clothing industry
- Clean rooms/food service industry
- Durable medical equipment/appliances industry
- Consulting industry

There are career opportunities in all of these subsectors. An aging population means there will be more need for long-term care expertise, both institutional and home based; bringing more people into the health care system through health care reform means there will be newer ways of delivering primary care, opening up new opportunities in both traditional physician practice management as well as cutting edge organizations.

HOSPITALS AND INTEGRATED CARE ORGANIZATIONS

Despite all of the movement toward ambulatory care over the last three decades, hospitals remain the largest single segment of the health care industry in terms of employment and in terms of where health care dollars are spent. In 2011, of the $2.7 trillion spent on health care in the United States, 33.4% was for some type of hospital care (*not* including long-term care). In second place was the physician services category at 21.3%, while pharmaceutical expenses represented 10.3% of all health care spending (CMSb, 2013). At the end of the current decade, in 2020, CMS estimates that hospital-related spending will dip to just above 30% (CMSb, 2013). At the same time, however, *total* health care spending will continue to escalate to $4.6 *trillion*. So while the hospitals' slice of the pie is diminishing slowly, the pie is growing. Furthermore, because baby boomers are starting to retire in increasing numbers every year, vacancies will be occurring in hospital management. This is encouraging if you are a job seeker.

Figure 3-1 provides a graphical representation of this expenditure distribution for the fiscal year 2010, along with the percentage distribution. The hospital remains "king of the hill" for where the expenditures are now, but as we progress toward new forms of clinical integration designed to provide more outpatient care and to provide earlier access to primary care, new organizations will emerge and the hospitals' share of this expenditure will be shared with new kinds of entities we are only beginning to see emerge today.

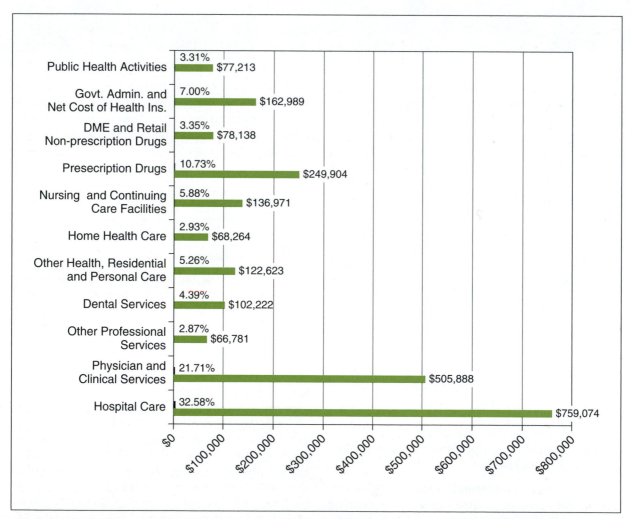

Figure 3-1 Fiscal year 2010 expenditure distribution and percentage distribution of health care industry.

Source: Adapted from U.S. Centers for Medicare and Medicaid Services, Office of the Actuary, "National Health Statistics Group." U.S. Centers for Medicare and Medicaid Services, Office of the Actuary, "National Health Statistics Group." http://www.cms.gov/NationalHealthExpendData/Internet release date: 09/30/2011

Hospitals are experiencing one of the highest rates of merger and acquisition on record—and, because of market pressures and the Patient Protection and Affordable Care Act (PPACA)—that trend shows no signs of abating (Mathews, 2011). Some of these hospital mergers are one to one; one to several; or even several to many, depending on local circumstances. There are three reasons for this wave of merger and acquisition activity: (1) to gain an advantageous bargaining position with insurance companies, (2) to eliminate duplication of costs, and (3) to obtain improved access to capital. The one that could be problematic for health administration students is the second factor, the elimination of duplicate costs. Those costs are generally in administrative areas. For example, if two hospitals decide to merge (or if one acquires the other), they generally will not need two administrative directors of radiology; or two administrative directors of general surgery, etc. So while the pie is growing faster than the hospital slice is shrinking is reason to be hopeful from a job perspective, the trend toward consolidation should also give one pause at least long enough to consider alternative avenues. (The other concern, of course, which is beyond the scope of this book, relates to the sustainability of the cost trend. PPACA was enacted, in part, to stem the tide of rising costs. Note that no one has—realistically—said it would be possible to *reduce* actual costs but only to slow the rate of increase.)

On paper, there are several reasons to believe hospitals will continue to be large employers. There is a retirement boom taking place in all industries in the United States and as hospitals are no exception, there is—and will be—a leadership shortage in the industry. Do not let the merger and acquisition activity scare you away from this field. Yes, consolidation does present some challenges, but as organizations change their focus from acute care to prevention, and as they lose leaders to retirement, they will need new talent and fresh eyes. The ability to create and implement facets of integrating clinical care across the continuum will be in big demand. Second, hospitals will continue to retain a significant percentage of all funds being spent on health care.

Conversely, there is an enormous degree of uncertainty given the changes in U.S. health policy in recent years. As of this writing, the implementation of PPACA is underway after being upheld—but weakened—by the U.S. Supreme Court. The long-term implications of this decision could have an extremely challenging impact on hospitals. In those states that have not yet decided to expand their Medicaid programs, a major pillar in the "universal coverage" envisioned by PPACA, then uncompensated care will continue to be a major financial concern for hospitals. Hospitals in states where Medicaid programs are expanding will be slightly better off as they will have fewer *private pay* or *charity care* patients in their beds. The uncertainty about the number of people who will actually be entering "the system" through PPACA and the general uncertainty about the economy, means there is a high degree of uncertainty about the future of small businesses and consumers, the main drivers of the U.S. economy. For those reasons, hospitals may be reluctant to make a commitment to young professionals seeking to begin their careers. (And for those of you seeking internships or residencies, do not be surprised to hear that "It is not in our budget.")

The other intriguing thing about hospitals is how they are changing their delivery strategies and how they will need to continue changing that strategy going forward. Hospitals are increasingly joining with physicians, or the other way around depending on your perspective, to provide a greater level of coordinated care, or clinically integrated care across the "continuum of care." Indeed, hospitals and insurance companies are working more closely together than ever before to promote common interests of reduced costs through better health (Blumenthal, 2011). In some cases, this is to form an accountable care organization (ACO) consistent with the requirements in PPACA. In other cases, this is a function of both market forces and the access to capital issue mentioned above. In either case, however, there will be a strong reliance on information technology (IT).

The need to pass patient information seamlessly between physician, hospital, insurance company, and such other providers as the patient may require is integrated care's *sine qua non*, the core—the very definition—of what it means to provide integrated care. Thus, if you have a strong information technology background, you are in a better position than others who may not have that particular skill or interest. The growth in health IT (HIT) jobs is expected to be very strong. One report said the number of HIT jobs will expand 21%, from 179,500 in 2010 to 217,200 in 2020. That number is to handle the dramatic growth in the amount of data that will need to be stored, secured, and transmitted as hospitals, physicians, and insurers connect in new and more significant ways (Xerox, 2012).

The mission of these integrated organizations will be strongly focused on preventive care, on improving the overall quality of care delivered, and the health status of the population those organizations serve. The financial incentives are shifting away from volume based to outcomes based. As a consequence, there will be a need for people who have a talent for integrating disparate missions and culture to a common purpose.

PHYSICIAN PRACTICE MANAGEMENT

Perhaps the one sector changing more than the hospital sector as a result of market forces and PPACA, among other legislative initiatives, is the physician practice. As of 2011, there were 230,187 physician offices in the United States (SKA, A Cegedim Company, 2012). Of those, 52.8% consisted of only one physician; 37.1% had two to five; 6.3% had six to nine and only 3.7% had more than 10 physicians. But the trend to look for in this is how many of those physician practice sites are or will become hospital-owned physician practices.

Medical Group Management Association (MGMA) reported in 2010 that hospital-owned practices were successful in attracting physicians to join them (MGMA, 2010). In that year, 65% of established physicians were placed in hospital-owned

services. Importantly, 49% of physicians hired out of their residency or fellowship joined hospital-owned practices. There are several reasons for this trend—somewhat similar to the underlying rationale for hospital mergers and acquisitions. First, the physicians feel they need a stronger voice in dealing with insurance companies and there is safety in numbers and with the hospital. Second, overhead continues to escalate while reimbursement levels stagnate. While hospitals want to eliminate duplication of some expenses, physicians are seeking to off-load at least some of their costs. Thus, they may turn to the hospital for an employment relationship. They may also opt to join together to eliminate, for example, the multiple offices of three providers in favor of a single location.

The upside is that as this sector congeals, particularly as the physicians join forces with the hospital to form integrated organizations, the need for professional management will grow. The physician practice formerly was a bit of a cottage industry. The man—and it was almost always a man—was the physician focused on seeing patients and his wife managed the business affairs of the office. This arrangement is still in place in many places in the United States. It is, however, like the family farm or the small community bank, a vanishing element of the health services landscape. As the character of practicing medicine migrates from being a cottage industry to becoming an active partner in integrated health services organizations managing population health in concert with other providers, the need for professional management will grow.

Administrators who can develop and maintain excellent relationships with physicians, whether through a hospital-owned practice or an independent physician practice, will bring tremendous value to their organizations. The differences in training and the differences in the professional expectations and cultures between administrators and physicians are substantial. Increasingly, there will be good management job opportunities as the alignment between hospitals and physicians improves. The anticipated—indeed mandated by PPACA—improvement in coordination of care means there will be a need for people who can help mediate the perspectives and coordinate the respective interests of both the hospital and the physicians.

HOME HEALTH CARE AND LONG-TERM CARE

There is no denying the aging of the population. As of 2010, the percent of the population over the age of 65 was 13.0%. By 2030, the mid-point of your career, that figure will be 19.3%. By 2050, about the time you begin to think of retirement, 20.2% of Americans will be over the age of 65 (Vincent & Velkrof, 2010). This will create both a tremendous opportunity for people interested in being in home health or long-term care, as well as an extraordinary burden on our society. Elders require more health care services owing to the stronger prevalence of chronic disease and assorted frailties associated with an older population (Federal Interagency on Aging-Related Statistics, 2012). For a visual representation, see Figure 3-2. You can see that the population from 2000 to 2010 has aged. Notice how the shaded portions—representing 2010—have grown over the outlined portions—representing 2000.

All of this portends an enormous demand for health services related to an elderly population. For both health and cost reasons, there will be an increasing emphasis on keeping the patient at home and out of an institutional setting (Ng, Harrison, & Kitchener, 2010). Consequently, growth in the home health industry is all but a foregone conclusion. Likewise, however, simply because the number of elders will be so significant, there will also be demand for increased capacity in long-term care facilities (Samala, Galindo, & Ciocon, 2011). In addition, the proportion of elderly who are dependent on others for care is likewise projected to grow (Vincent & Velkrof, 2010).

Consider, for example, that there are more than 12,000 Medicare-certified home health agencies and nearly 8,000 more that are not but that provide home-based health care (HomeHealthCareAgencies, 2013).

Not only will the proportion of the population be older, thereby necessitating a greater degree of health care services intended for them, but we will continue to live longer, thus compounding the demand for age-appropriate services. Concomitantly, CMS projects increased spending for both Medicare and Medicaid, both of which fund health care services for the elderly (CMSb, 2010).

A rapidly growing—perhaps the most rapidly growing—segment of the health care market is *assisted living*. This is a form of a retirement community that often is a precursor to a skilled nursing home. Indeed, often this is the entry to a continuing care retirement community.

Assisted living generally provides a retiree with congregate housing, a social setting, assistance at a minimal level for activities of daily living, and an environment that is safe, clean, and amenable to the resident's lifestyle. This is a form of retirement living that is far less restrictive than a nursing home and provides a level of care that is attentive for things like overseeing the administration of medications, arranging social events and outings, and providing either stand-by or hands-on assistance for things like dressing, bathing, transferring, toileting, or showering. The resident has complete freedom to come and go to the extent they are able. What makes this attractive for elderly people who are still active and cognitively able is that they can interact with others and be as mobile as they are capable. At the same time, should their physical and/or mental condition deteriorate, they are generally not far from more intensive care. As baby boomers retire at the rate of approximately 10,000 per day, this segment of the industry will continue to grow rapidly and represents a significant professional opportunity for would-be managers.

MANAGED CARE PLANS AND INSURANCE COMPANIES

For people interested in the delivery of health care services, this may be considered the "dark side." In fact, however, the financing of the delivery of health care services is vital. Indeed, the financing of health care is nothing less than the allocation of critical resources to deliver health services. There is increasing alignment taking place between the finance and

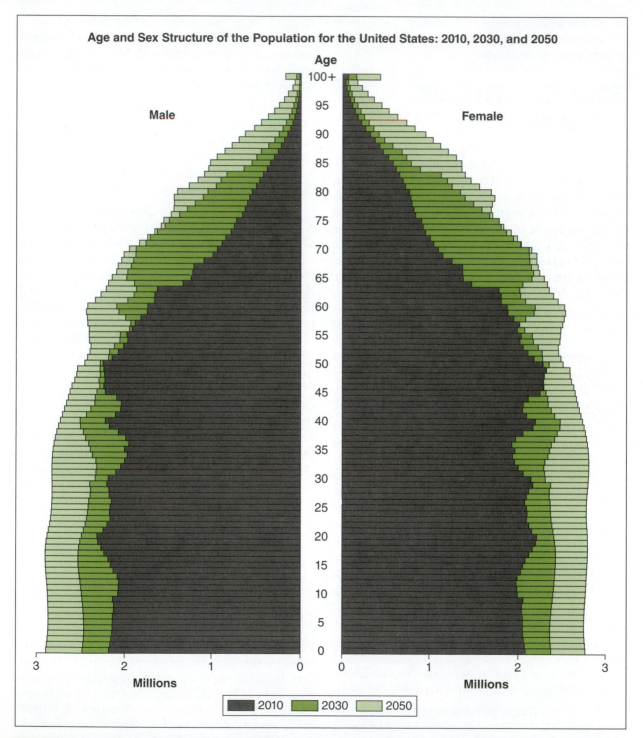

Figure 3-2 Age and sex structure of the population for the United States: 2010, 2030, and 2050.

Source: U.S. Census Bureau, 2008

delivery sectors. Note that some of the most success-ful health care organizations in the United States have health plans associated with the delivery of their health services: Kaiser, UPMC, Geisinger, Group Health of Puget Sound, for example. Consider that there is an increasing number of alignments between insurance organizations and hospitals, such as the West Penn Allegheny and Highmark Blue Cross/ Blue Shield relationship in Pittsburgh (Pennsylvania Insurance Department, 2013). Indeed, one com-mentator has gone so far as to suggest *insurance* as such will not exist in the future, but rather become a part of integrated enterprises called accountable care organizations (Emanuel, 2012). Whether that ever really happens, what *will* remain is a need to have people who understand financing health care and managing risk. Even if it is not called *insurance*, there will still be a need for people associated with the financing of health care services.

PHARMACEUTICALS

The future of the pharmaceutical industry would seem to be very positive. The trend in health care is away from the in-patient setting, focusing increasingly on providing preventive and chronic disease manage-ment in ambulatory settings. Part of that migration is possible because of the growth in the spectrum of prescription drugs to effectively provide care.

But, like other sectors of the health care industry, this sector, too will confront dramatic changes. Some of that change will come about because patents on some of the major blockbuster drugs either have recently expired or will expire in the near future. This paves the way for generic drug competition. Second, the science of blockbuster drugs is not what it once was: There are few known major new drugs in the development pipe-line. Finally, even though use of drugs may represent a net cost savings to the health care system, overall cost containment efforts will impact the pharmaceutical industry (Kandybin & Genova, 2012; Silverman, 2012).

While the industry may change its model from simply "selling the pill" to being measured based on outcomes performance, the fact remains that it will also enjoy growing markets. In the United States, as many as 37 million new people will be insured in the

wake of health care reform. These are all prospec-tive customers for the pharmaceutical industry—customers who will have insurance to pay for many of the prescription drug needs.

THE PROVIDER SUPPORT SECTOR

While this sector does not provide direct care and it does not arrange the financing of health care, the groups of companies in this category provide valuable services to health service organizations and patients alike. We do not often think of companies such as General Electric or Siemens as having much to do with health care ser-vices. To the contrary, they manufacture imaging devices and provide other services to health services organiza-tions that are indispensable. And there are several other groups that fall into this category as well. There are a host of these companies, including ARAMARK and Sodexho, that provide equipment, services, and main-tenance to hospitals and health care services organi-zations that keep those organizations running. These services range from food service, laundry services, build-ing maintenance, to biomedical repair and update. All of these things are essential to a successful health care organization and none of them is a luxury.

Consulting

This is another avenue into health care. While con-sultants do not have anything to do—directly—with the delivery of health care services, they perform a wide variety of invaluable services to those who do. This option is, however, often less sedentary than other kinds of careers in health care. Consultants frequently travel. And depending on the assignment, that can mean living in temporary quarters from Monday to Thursday, returning home for the week-ends on Friday. Other times, there can be downtime in the office when business is slow. Then there are long hours with your head stuck in a computer mon-itor looking at spreadsheets. All of this, of course, depends on the type of consulting firm and the type of assignment. Revenue cycle management is a major source of consulting work. Strategic planning, needs assessments, service line development, developing medical staff plans, installing and training electronic medical record systems, and assessments leading to restructuring to become more effective or efficient, are all tasks frequently performed by consultants.

One upside of starting a career as a consultant is that you can gain terrific experience. You also get to work in a variety of organizations—large and small; urban and rural; teaching and nonteaching venues, and the like. This kind of experience helps one develop a perspective about what kind of organization *they* would like to join. One downside is that you can get tagged as someone who has never had to *implement* any decisions, but rather come to town, make a recommendation, and then disappear before the recommendation becomes reality. Indeed, the decisions look a bit different from the inside—where the work needs to be done to carry them out—than on the outside—where the one doing the recommending is not responsible for living with the consequences. You can overcome this— like everything else, it is all up to you.

You should check out the American Association of Healthcare Consultants for starters. This is a relatively small sampling of the many, many firms that provide a wide range of services to health care providers (AAHC, 2011).

Medical Equipment, Instruments, and Appliances

The traditional definition of this term related mostly to medical imaging devices or machines used in viewing or assessing unusual changes or things in the body. The contemporary use of the term includes biomedical engineering—engineers that work hand-in-hand with physicians to devise artificial limbs and other prostheses that actually relate to the nervous system of the human body, providing patients some new degree of functionality they would not be able to achieve with a static prosthesis. If you are reading *this* book, chances are good that you are not an engineer. The point in mentioning this part of the health care industry is to help you see another career avenue. You do not need to be a physician or an engineer to work in a company like this. Granted, some technical background would be helpful, but companies like this still need managers, compliance officers, client support personnel, and

the like. This segment of the industry has grown at a rapid pace since the 1980s. University business collaborations have spurred the development of new devices intended to extend the level of care delivered to the patients (DeVol, Bedroussian, & Yeo, 2011). Some of the industry leaders are as follows: GE Healthcare, Siemens, Amgen, Genentech, Genzyme, Gilead Science, and Novartis—and there are literally thousands more.

There are companies that provide all manner of services to hospitals. When you think of a company like ARAMARK, for example, you generally think food services. It is true that they provide that service, but they do a host of other services in support of hospitals such as housekeeping and biomedical. Hospitals are learning that in many cases it is less expensive to outsource a service than to build internal capacity to run it. What this means from your perspective is that there are health care-related career opportunities in many companies like ARAMARK, Sodexho, and others that provide not only food service, but offer a wide variety of support services to hospitals.

CONCLUSION

When it comes to finding a career in health care, there are literally thousands of possibilities. While we often think only of hospitals or long-term care or physician practice management, there are many other kinds of organizations that play key roles in the delivery of health care services in the United States. This chapter has been only an introduction to the many nontraditional venues in which you might find career fulfillment. The challenge for you is to conduct a search—a very thorough search—of all the kinds of organizations that are engaged in the delivery of health care services.

Previously, this book focused on how to help you identify yourself so you can find a proper fit for your skills, talents, and interests in the context of a career-launching job. Here, you have read about a few ideas about where to look. In the remainder of the text, you will find ways to execute your job search that will result in success.

Observations from the Professionals

Why You Should Use Career Services on Your Campus

Jill Pletcher serves as the Director of Career Services at Wichita State University in Wichita, KS. Wichita State is Kansas' only urban-serving university and has an enrollment of 15,000 students.

You are close to earning your degree. You have learned a tremendous amount about your field of study—from professors and instructors, from textbooks, practicums, internships, and other hands-on experiences. You are ready and eager to move into a professional position.

Next step: job search.
Let the fun begin.
On the plus side, there is a multitude of people who can be helpful with what can be a long, unfamiliar, ever-changing, and frustrating process:

- Professors/instructors
  In addition to what you have learned from them in classes, they often have professional and community connections that may be helpful in generating job leads.

- Practicum/internship supervisors
  Seeing students' qualities and capabilities first-hand may give them an advantage when they have openings within their organizations.

- Friends and family members
  Even if they do not know of job openings, they may know of someone who does or someone who could help you make appropriate connections.

- Career services professionals
  Career services professionals are like a coach—they cannot play the job search game for you (i.e., find you a job), but they can provide great strategies to help you sharpen your game.

This book covers a broad range of topics directly applicable to your professional development. Sometimes it is helpful, however, to talk with someone about how those guidelines apply to your particular circumstances. This is where a career services professional can be beneficial. For example, I have worked with students who have read multiple resources about how to write a resume, including ones put out by our office. But their unique circumstances may not have been covered. Or when I review the draft they have created, I may see additional or alternate ways for them to highlight their qualifications. Recommendations are tailored to their particular situation, not just résumés in general.

Although services may vary by campus, career services professionals often offer the following types of assistance:

Career counseling
Students utilize career counseling services for a variety of reasons, including:

Choosing between several majors of interest

Changing majors because an initial choice was not a good fit

Gauging options for careers within a given major. This may involve doing informational interviews with professionals for the purpose of understanding what their day-to-day work is really like. It may also include shadowing professionals to confirm career interests.

Resume and cover letter reviews
Benefits include the following:

- An experienced set of eyes to proofread for proper punctuation, grammar, spelling, and clarity
- A fresh perspective from someone who does not already know you
- Seeing your materials through the eyes of potential employers. Most career services professionals have ongoing contact with employers in order to remain up to date with current hiring practices. This includes preferred résumé formats and length, use of key words, online applications and applicant tracking systems, volume of applicants, and what helps applicants get noticed for the *right* reasons.

Interview preparation and mock interview(s)
Benefits include the following:

- Learning how to research an employer
- Clarifying what to take with you, how early to arrive, and including *everyone* you meet as part of the interview process
- Presenting yourself professionally, including introductions, handshakes, and eye contact
- Confirming that your selected attire is appropriate
- Understanding types of interview questions most frequently asked and how to prepare for them
- Practicing out loud versus just thinking through what you might say

- Preparing appropriate questions to ask the interviewer
- Having the opportunity to receive candid feedback about your mannerisms, questions, and responses

Interview follow-up
Benefits include the following:

- Understanding when and how to follow up after an interview
- Weighing how well a specific position fits you
- Learning if/when/how to negotiate a salary offer
- Understanding your options if you receive multiple offers from different employers

Additional suggestions

- Get acquainted early on with your career services professionals so they can get to know you and can keep an eye out for resources and opportunities that pertain to your career objectives
- Ask if there is someone in the career services office with a particular expertise in health care employment
- Bring copies of the position listing(s) for which you are applying with you to your appointment. That will help your career advisor help you tailor your materials to those positions
- Do multiple mock interviews with different career services staff members
- Request the opportunity to do mock interviews with local employers

EXERCISES

3-1. Develop a list of all the *different kinds* of hospitals you can find. Include all the specialty hospitals.

3-2. Find a trade journal article on emerging organizational structures in health care. Write a short (two or three pages) paper on the impact of clinical integration on management.

3-3. Make a list of all the different kinds of organizations you can find that claim to be related to providing health care services.

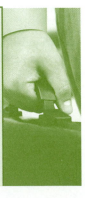

BIBLIOGRAPHY

AAHC. (2011). *Home: American Association of Healthcare Consultants*. Retrieved February 12, 2012, from AAHC website: http://www.aahc.net/

Blumenthal, R. G. (2011, October 30). *Merger Wave Hits Health Care*. Retrieved April 23, 2012, from *The Wall Street Journal*: http://online.wsj.com

CMSa. (2012, January 6). *National Health Expenditure Data*. Retrieved February 8, 2012, from CMS website: https://www.cms.gov/NationalHealthExpendData/25_NHE_Fact_Sheet.asp

CMSb. (2010). *National Health Expenditure Projections*. Retrieved March 30, 2013, from Centers for Medicare and Medicaid Services: https://www.cms.gov

CMSb. (2013,). *Research-Statistics-Data-and Systems*. Retrieved February 20, 2014, from CMS.GOV: https://www.cms.gov/Research-Statistics-Data-and-Systems/Statistics-Trends-and-Reports/NationalHealthExpendData/Downloads/PieChartSourcesExpenditures2010.pdf

DeVol, R., Bedroussian, A., & Yeo, B. (2011, September 22). *The Global Biomedical Industry: Preserving US Leadership*. Retrieved February 11, 2012, from Milken Institute website: http://www.milkeninstitute.org/publications/publications.taf?function=detail&ID=38801285&cat=resrep

Emanuel, E. J. (2012, January 30). *Opinionator Blog*. Retrieved February 8, 2012, from *New York Times*: http://opinionator.blogs.nytimes.com/2012/01/30the-end-of-helath-insurance-companies

Federal Interagency on Aging-Related Statistics. (2012). *Older Americans 2012: Key Indicators of Well Being*. Retrieved March 4, 2013, from Agingstats.gov: http://www.agingstats.gov/Main_Site/Data/2012_Documents/docs/EntireChartbook.pdf

HomeHealthCareAgencies. (2013). Retrieved April 3, 2013, from HomeHealthCareAgencies.com: http://www.homehealthcareagencies.com/

Kandybin, A., & Genova, V. (2012, February 28). *Big Pharma's Uncertain Future*. Retrieved April 3, 2013, from Strategy + Business: http://m.strategy-business.com/

Keckley, P., & Bigalke, J. (2011). *2012 Outlook on Helath Care, Life Sciences and Government*. Retrieved February 12, 2012, from Deloitte: http://www.deloitte.com/view/en_US/us/Insights/hot-topics/2012-industry-outlook/bf99582cad7c3310VgnVCM2000001b56f00aRCRD.htm

Mathews, A. W. (2011, December 12). *The Future of Healthcare*. Retrieved April 23, 2012, from WSJ.COM: http://online.wsj.com/article/SB100014240529702043190045770845553869990554.html

MGMA. (2010, June 3). *Press Releases*. Retrieved April 24, 2012, from www.MGMA.COM: http://www.mgma.com/press/default.aspx?id=33777

Ng, T., Harrison, C., & Kitchener, M. (2010). Medicare and Medicaid in Long Term Care. *Helath Affairs*, 22–28.

Pennsylvania Insurance Department. (2013, January 23). *Pennsylvania Insurance Department*. Retrieved March 20, 2013, from State of Pennsylvania: http://www.portal.state.pa.us

Samala, R., Galindo, D., & Ciocon, J. (2011). Transitioning Nursing Home Patients with Demential to Hospice Care. *Annals of Long Term Care: Clinical Care and Aging*, 41–47.

Silverman, E. (2012, September 25). *And the Crystal Ball Says The Pharma Future is Improving*. Retrieved April 3, 2013, from Forbes.com: www.forbes.com

SKA, A Cegedim Company. (2012, February 12). *SKA Live Counts*. Retrieved April 24, 2012, from Live Counts: http://www.skalivecounts.com/

Vincent, G. K., & Velkrof, V. A. (2010, May). *The Next Four Decades, The Older Population in the United States: 2010 to 2050*. Washington, D.C.: U.S. Census Bureau.

Xerox. (2012, April 10). *The Future of Health Care*. Retrieved April 23, 2012, from The Healthcare Blog: http://thehealthcareblog.com/files

Chapter 4

It Is Not Only WHAT You Know: Networking and Learning More

Networking is a critically important part of your career development. Perhaps you have heard the expression that luck is nothing more than the meeting of opportunity and preparation. Networking is in large measure about creating opportunity for you in your career advancement. This is not about putting on a false front *pretending* to take an interest in others. The approach to this should be one of genuine interest: interest in the work of others; interest in learning more about the health care industry; interest in learning more about the world in general from the others' points of view; and certainly not the least, interest in learning how you can help others. In advancing that curiosity, networking is also about preparation: It is just another way of continuing on the path of being a lifelong learner. Thus, networking is doubly important in the development of your career.

At the end of this chapter, you will be able to identify networking opportunities; understand that networking is more than a handshake and an exchange of business cards; understand the importance of professional associations; and identify yourself and your interests in a brief "elevator speech."

WHAT IS NETWORKING?

Networking is the art of taking a professional interest in the lives of others while sharing some parts of yourself as well. Remember the guy in Chapter 2 who went up to the speaker and said "Great job; do you take interns because I need one?" This is exactly antithetical to what networking is really about.

First, be genuine. Throughout this text you have found, and will find, that when you do *anything* to represent yourself, you should, above all, *be* yourself. It is counterproductive, not to mention unethical, to represent yourself as something you are not. Let us suppose you are at a national professional conference, for example, and you meet a CFO and have a terrific conversation with him. You have the feeling there could be a career with the organization he has described for you as fast growing and dynamic. Trying to impress him, you let him believe you are a terrific financial analyst, when, in fact, your quantitative skills are so poor you have anxiety attacks every time you open Excel. The fact is your real passion is in supply chain management; so why not tell him? There may still be career opportunities in his organization. Frankly, it does not matter because the real purpose of your conversation with him was to learn more about his organization and his role in it. They may have a suitable opening for you in a year or two, or perhaps three. Your acquaintanceship with the CFO will still have a positive impact, especially if you have stayed in touch in the intervening years. (This introduces the notion of the "fit" you should be looking for as you undertake your job search, discussed at greater length later in Chapter 10.)

The point here is simple: Be yourself. If you represent yourself as who you are and why you are pointing in a particular direction, then a process that is already hard enough (especially if you are an introvert) becomes just a slight bit easier. When you have that conversation with the CFO, remember it is not just about you getting a job; it is about learning more regarding the industry, his organization, and him.

One of the benefits of the networking process is that you will build a large contact file in your smartphone or computer. The larger the list in the planner, the more likely it is that you will expedite the job searching process, whether it is a voluntary or an involuntary move, an internship, residency, fellowship, or first job.

You will find in the "Observations from the Professionals" box some real life examples about why networking is so important, more about how to do it, and most importantly, that it is not so much about you as it is about learning and helping others.

PROFESSIONAL MEETINGS

Professional meetings are the *sine qua non* with regard to networking. One of the primary reasons these things take place is to give professionals an opportunity to get to know one another and learn from one another. Whether you are an undergrad or an MHA student, these meetings can be very important for you. Regardless of what your interest in the field is, whether you aspire to run a hospital, a medical practice, or a long-term care facility (or other), you can—and should—find a professional association to join. Then attend the annual meeting and any regional meetings you can find.

No one has the holy grail on how to manage a health care organization. Everyone is aspiring to be better. Leaders and managers set goals, achieve them, and then set new goals. In the process, one may develop a pretty good idea for managing, say, ER wait times. As a service to the profession, that person may submit a proposal to present at the next annual convention of their professional group. You attend because you want to be a life-long learner and

grow professionally and because, as an intern, you studied your hospital's ER wait times only to find they are abysmal, you go to this session. You learn a few things and share them with your former preceptor. This seems pretty simple, but the point is this is but one way of how professional education takes place. The purpose of professional meetings (either regionally or nationally) is to share ideas about what works and what does not work. In the process, people who have similar interests meet one another and develop a collegial or professional relationship. It is the give and take of good ideas that helps drive continual improvement.

At professional meetings, not only is there the give and take of formal educational sessions described above, but there are usually multiple opportunities to meet others informally. If there is an exhibit hall, go check it out. Walk around and see what you can learn from the exhibits. At the same time, you will have the opportunity to talk with people supporting the exhibits as well as with other professionals doing the same thing. Strike up a conversation with some of these folks; the exhibits give you a perfect excuse to say something as you and the fellow wandering professional have just each taken at least a cursory interest in the same thing. Then you can enlarge the conversation to the meeting itself and by asking more about them and their organization. Be sure to exchange business cards. Complete Exercise 4-1 before moving on to the rest of the chapter.

Usually, it is the large, national meetings that have an exhibit room. Other smaller meetings may not. Whether the meeting is a large national conference or a small regional conference, chances are there will be a lunch or dinner. Sit at a table where you do not know anyone. Even better, if you are with a friend, then the two of you sit together and help each other get to know everyone else at the table. Do *not* just talk to each other because that is comfortable for you. Get beyond your comfort zone. The same general concepts apply. Be curious. Ask your dining partners questions about their organization or their own career. Talk about one of the presentations you attended; ask them about one *they* attended. Be sure to exchange business cards as well. Complete Exercise 4-2 before moving on to the rest of the chapter.

And one thing that is *always* a part of a professional meeting is the reception. Here, too, you can find people, start a conversation and develop an acquaintanceship. Again, be curious; seek to understand them and what they do and exchange business cards.

Of course, the reception presents a unique dynamic: the consumption of alcohol. As a student, it is best if you do not drink at all at these events. But if you are of legal age and make the choice to have an alcoholic beverage, be *moderate* in your consumption. Moderate in this setting is one (normal size) drink. A handy rule for this is "one and done." There are a couple of reasons for either abstaining or drinking in moderation. First, the purpose of being there is to meet people, get acquainted, and learn something. It will be helpful to you later if you actually remember the people you have met and the gist of the conversations you have had. Whether you believe or not, it is true that alcohol impairs your memory (White, 2004). Second, however, we are back to Chapter 2—you never get a second chance to make a first impression. If your idea is to take advantage of the free booze and get tanked, what kind of impression are you making? Again, whether you believe it or not, alcohol does affect your behavior (Abroms, Fillmore, & Marczinski, 2003). Let us just say there are three phases of getting drunk: (1) you think you are rich and famous; (2) you think you are bulletproof; and (3) you think you are invisible. You are, of course, none of those things. Most folks will probably start to behave as if they are "rich and famous" if they have more than one drink. If you think you want to be that, or bulletproof, or invisible, leave the reception. You will not help yourself by staying. And, frankly, you will not help yourself by leaving and drinking until you enter one of these fictional conditions either, but at least you might be able to preserve a fraction of a professional image. Your best choice is to abstain; the second best choice is to limit yourself to one drink. There are no good choices after that. Keep your eye on the prize: professional growth through an expanding network of friends and acquaintances.

NETWORKING RESOURCES AND IDEAS

There are a lot of places to look for new connections and new entrées to the industry. There certainly is nothing wrong with asking family and friends if they know someone with whom you can talk about what it is like to be in the health care field. If you have an aunt who is the CEO of a community hospital, take advantage of that family connection, call on her to learn about what her work is like and what it took for her to earn that level of success. Similarly, if a family friend is the administrative director of surgery for the local academic medical center, there is nothing wrong with making arrangements to shadow him to learn about his work. One of the things about health care is that nearly everyone in a leadership position has benefited from the help or mentorship of someone else and nearly all of them are willing, if not anxious, to pay it back. One characteristic we all seem to have at some level is that we are caregivers. It is a part of the profession.

Beyond family and friends, however, there are a multitude of other resources available to you. First and foremost, the members of the faculty in your program are possible networking resources. Remember in the first chapter the discussion about how virtually anyone can be a reference? Faculty members are often called by organizations and alumni looking for good people. It would be helpful if they could mention you on those occasions; perhaps even more helpful if they would pick up the phone and make a call to someone on your behalf. They can help get you started networking by providing you an entrée to an alum or two or to an organization.

Alumni can be of help. Your program may have an active student—alumni mentor program or something similar. If so, become active in it. Get acquainted with some of your program's alumni.

These are people who can help you start the networking process when the time comes for you to undertake your job search. Again, someone probably helped them, so they are likely more than willing to help you so do not be shy about asking for help.

Your university probably has a career services office. This, too, can be a valuable resource for finding possible networking beginnings. The professionals who work in these offices make it their business to stay in touch with a wide variety of businesses and industries and are knowledgeable about advising students. They can provide you personalized assistance in finding a path to get started as you begin your professional career.

Finally, professional associations frequently maintain job sites and bulletin boards where prospective employees and employers can exchange information. You can often post your information on the site and perhaps make a connection to start interviewing or networking through that option. There are some links to several professional associations at the end of the chapter.

Of course, you can find ways to meet individuals, but what is it you want from them. You cannot simply make an appointment, show up, be shown into the office by the secretary, shake hands, plop yourself down in the chair, and say "'S'sup; I was wonderin' if you had a job for me." A more subtle, longer-term approach might be better, which brings us to "the informational interview."

INFORMATIONAL INTERVIEWS

If you consider professional gatherings as some kind of "wholesale networking," then the informational interview is retail: This is one-on-one interview and is an incredibly effective tool. While being incredibly effective, it can also seem intimidating.

Where to start? There are many ways to get started. You might have an aunt who is the administrator of a group practice, or an uncle who is an executive with a hospital. Perhaps a friend of your parents is

in health care, or a neighbor. In addition, someone you meet at a professional gathering is a good place to start. You have already met them; you have their contact information because you exchanged business cards. If you do not have anyone in these categories, then consider calling on the guest speaker in class or the guest speaker at your student club.

Remember the two people in Chapter 2: the guy who exhibits exactly the wrong thing to do and the one who "gets" it? Part—only part—of the reason you want to be more like the second person in that scene is because you might want to do this very thing. Notice the smart guy in that example gave the speaker his business card and said he would like to meet with him sometime. He already set up to open the door for this experience. If you did the right thing at the professional meeting, you have several opportunities: people you met in the exhibit hall; people you met at lunch or dinner; and, of course, people you met at the reception.

Having identified someone you think is interesting and might be willing to give you some time to help you learn more, the next step is to reach out to them. If you have their business card, you have a choice to make: Use the e-mail address on the card and approach the person directly, or call the phone number and talk to an assistant. This is a choice you make partly on your "feel" for the conversation you had and partly on the rank of the person on whom you are focused for this purpose. If you had a really terrific conversation with someone who is an administrative director or a program manager or something similar, then e-mailing directly to that person is likely the best bet. If you had a very brief, casual conversation with a CEO or COO then calling and talking to the assistant is likely the smart move. There are a couple of reasons for this: First, someone at that level probably does not keep their own calendar. Second, keep in mind the likely age difference here; if it was just a quick, casual conversation, the recipient of the e-mail might be more likely to see the e-mail as a bit of a bother since he or she will then need to respond to you and copy his or her assistant so they can get you scheduled. For some, even most perhaps, this is not a big deal. For the relative few, however, it might be a small negative before you even get to the office door. Just to be clear, if you *do* decide to e-mail the COO or CEO, it is *not* "Dear First Name." It is Dear "Dr./Mr./Ms. Last name."

If you call the assistant, you do run the risk that they are some kind of Praetorian Guard dog whose job it is to keep the riffraff like you out of the office and not in the boss's way. But there is risk no matter which way you go, so do not let it stop you. When you call the assistant, you will need to explain who you are, when you met the boss, perhaps a bit of the conversation you had with the boss, and ask for some time to see him or her. Put on your very best manners and pleasant voice in making this request. This person, too, is a professional. They help the boss set priorities because they help manage his or her time. They likely are a confidant. You do not want this person going to the boss and saying, "She seemed a bit uppity on the phone. Kind of entitled, I think." Even if you are successful in getting the meeting scheduled, the boss is now predisposed to see you in that light and look for evidence that the assistant described. The assistant, as the old saying goes, poisoned the well. The meeting will likely be nothing more than an exchange of pleasantries when you are interested in getting a more in-depth look at the health care industry, this organization, and this person. It costs nothing to engage with that assistant in a positive, mannerly way.

So, e-mail or call, the choice is yours. There are some minor risks associated with either approach, but on balance those are petty things that should not deter you from getting in the door to see this person.

What to Talk about When You Are There

The objective of the informational interview is not, in the short term, to help you get a job. This is an opportunity to get to know more about the health care industry from the perspective of someone actually doing the job. You can also learn more about the organization you are visiting as well as the person herself. And all of this has *tremendous* value. Of course, when you get in the office, the conversation should begin with something to the effect "Thank you for taking the time to see me. I am anxious to learn more about health care and I am grateful you would take the time to help me." It is OK to be a bit of a supplicant here—you are. Of course, these should be your own words, so you can replace *health care* with whatever subspecialty of the person with whom you are speaking. From there, it is simply a matter of being genuinely curious and listening. There is a reason we have two ears and one mouth: Use them in about the same proportion.

You should be prepared before going to make this visit. Review the organization's website. What kind of service(s) does it provide? Has it won any noteworthy awards? This research does not have to be as in depth as it would if you were seeking a job or an internship, but you should have enough of an idea about what is going on to ask intelligent questions about the organization itself.

Questions you might ask are:

- "What do you think are the most significant issues in health care today?"
- "How is (your organization) dealing with that issue?"
- "What is the most significant challenge you face at (your organization)?"
- "How did you prepare for your position? What is your background?"

Now here is the hard part. *Listen*—actively—to the answers. Relate something your host has said to something you studied in class. This is not solely an interview, but a *conversation*. Demonstrate that you (a) heard what was said and (b) have learned some things and can apply them to the real world. When she says that "transitioning to population-based reimbursement methodologies" is the most significant issue in health care, do *not* sit there with your mouth agape. Make an observation and follow up: "We learned that issue is part of the accountable care mandate in health care reform in my classes; how is this impacting (your organization)?"

Remember, networking is both *opportunity* and *preparation*. You contribute to your preparation by listening to, and learning from, the answers to your questions. You contribute to the opportunity by demonstrating you have some degree of understanding what your host is saying.

Do not be afraid of, or intimidated, by this process. First, most administrators (especially the good ones) are willing to help. Chances are someone helped them and they have an instinct to give back. Second, if this sort of thing makes you uncomfortable, well, get over it. As you move through your career, hopefully ascending to the next level every few years, you will find that you will be required to do things you do not know how to do; be required to know things you do not know; and be required to solve problems you do not know how to solve. All of these things will make you uncomfortable and that is OK. What will be necessary is for you to learn *how* to do things you do not know how to do; *learn* the things you do not know; and *figure out* how to solve the problem you do not know how to solve. In other words, be confident and have faith in yourself. Do not be cocky, but understand that life is a journey of learning and growth. Just like those episodes in your career described above, networking is something you need to learn how to do. Trust in yourself that your academic preparation and the preparation of this book will provide the tools you need to have an interesting conversation with someone from whom you can learn a great deal.

CO-CURRICULAR ACTIVITIES

These, too, represent excellent networking opportunities. Remember that your fellow students are the beginning of your professional network. In addition, when your club takes a field trip or has a guest speaker, it is yet another opportunity to make a first impression. All the things mentioned in this chapter have application in this particular setting. Dress appropriately. Be considerate of the speaker's or host's time. Ask good questions.

Treat this as you would a professional conference. Indeed, it is the practice ground for that very thing. Use it and learn from it.

ELECTRONIC NETWORKING

Chapter 2 addressed this partly in the context of what kind of content should *not* be on your Facebook page and about how to use social media to promote your identity. LinkedIn has particular application here.

As you meet professionals in the field, in whatever venue, search for them on LinkedIn. If you have met them, go ahead and ask to be a *connection*. Again, do not be shy: The most they can do is hit the *ignore* button. Most won't.

At the same time, it is helpful if you build an *electronic résumé* on your LinkedIn page as mentioned in Chapter 2.

This gets to a couple of other points discussed at greater depth elsewhere in the book: (1) you want to have good projects in your internship, something from which you can show results and (2) use active verbs to present what you did (see Chapter 6). It is *not* important that you were an intern at Biggest-Best Hospital System; it *is* important to demonstrate what you did in that role.

Often the first thing someone will do when they get a request to connect on LinkedIn is to look at the profile of the person making the request. So when the CEO of Biggest-Best Hospital System speaks to the local ACHE club and gets a subsequent request from this person to connect, what does he see? You want material that describes that you can apply your knowledge to the real world. This is why you need good projects in your internship(s).

Marry this to the notion of putting your LinkedIn page as a link in the signature block of your e-mail. Note how I have used LinkedIn in my e-mail signature block in Figure 4-1.

Now, every time you send someone an e-mail, you are sending them a virtual résumé. If you have prepared it well by getting good experiences and displaying them well, you are, in effect, marketing yourself. Using LinkedIn as a kind of marketing résumé is appropriate at any educational or professional level, so whether you are an undergrad or an MHA student

Michael R. Meacham, JD, MPH

Associate Professor
Department of Healthcare Leadership and Management
Medical University of South Carolina
151-B Rutledge MSC 962
Charleston, SC 29425
(843) 792-5402
Fax: (843) 792-3327

Figure 4-1 An example of an e-mail signature line with a link to the author's LinkedIn profile.

or a full-time, high-level professional, you can list interesting things under "Experience." Literally, take the detail from your résumé and put it on LinkedIn.

STARTING A CONVERSATION AND THE "ELEVATOR SPEECH"

For some people this is quite difficult. For the more extraverted among us, they never met a stranger and have no problem striking up a conversation with anyone. It really does not take a lot to begin a conversation at a networking event. Questions are a good way to start, like the examples earlier in this chapter. Remember, if you are nervous about this sort of thing, you are most certainly not alone. Look around the room; you will see at least one person who looks to be alone and not interacting. Walk up to that person: "Have you ever been to this convention before?" is a good way to get started.

It may help those who are a bit introverted—actually it can help everyone—to prepare somewhat. Think ahead of time of a couple of questions you can ask: "How did you get started in your career?" or "Tell me more about your organization." Frankly, it is always a good idea at these kinds of meetings and events to ask questions. People generally feel good talking about themselves or their organizations.

It always helps to smile. It will help people approach you and it will make you less threatening if you approach them. You do not need to walk around with a grin like the Cheshire cat from *Alice in Wonderland*, but a good smile conveys warmth and openness, standing with a frown, not so much.

It also helps to do this with a friend. Again, do not stand against the wall talking to each other. You already believe in each other. It is easier to mingle in crowds and approach strangers if you do it with someone. You can introduce each other to help remove the burden of doing it all yourself.

Much of this depends on the context. Assuming you are at a professional meeting, either a regional or national conference, the process is more general than the informational interview discussed above. So opening lines like: "I really enjoyed the session on ("x" topic). Did you go to that one?" And if "yes," then you have something specific to discuss. If the answer is "no" you can follow up with "What was the most interesting session you attended?" If you are a first-time attendee at a conference, it is most certainly appropriate to say so and ask for some suggestions about the event. Try something like: "I have never been to this meeting before, can you give me some advice about the best sessions or speakers?"

If you want to ask for advice on a different level perhaps, "I will be completing my degree this semester and wonder what it would be like to work at your organization. Can you tell me a little bit about it?" Or, "I am a student in health administration and am curious about (fill in a specialty that (a) genuinely interests you and (b) the other person will know something about). Can you give me some advice?"

If you have had a good conversation with someone, but it is time to move on for whatever reason, try to find a way to follow up: "This has been a great conversation and I would love to have an opportunity to talk some more. Would it be OK for me to contact you in the near future to schedule a meeting so we could continue our conversation?" (This is basically a request for an "informational interview" discussed above. Do you see how these experiences can build on one another?)

In the course of all of this, naturally, someone is going to say something like "Tell me about yourself." For this, you need to be prepared. It will not do to stand there and break out in a cold sweat mumbling something about being a student at Big Time State University. By the same token, this statement was not an invitation for you to share intimate details of your life's story and that you think you are a future leader of the Western world. A balanced effort here would be appropriate. Many refer to this as the "elevator speech." Some say the term comes from the days of Internet developers seeking venture capital and would only have a brief time on an elevator to explain to a venture capitalist why they should invest in this particular enterprise. Some say it came from the idea that a CEO is on an elevator with a job candidate in an unplanned meeting and says, "Tell me about yourself." There simply is not a great deal of time to get in the key points. Even if your exchange is not on an elevator, you should get the key points out in a relatively short period of time, about 30 seconds or so.

What do you say? Well, what is important to you? Go back to Chapter 1 and review the exercises. Encapsulate (a) your university status; (b) your career interests; (c) why that interest, what your passion is; (d) what are your strengths; (e) how others would describe you; and (f) how you want to develop professionally. Ideally, you should be able to mention all this in a conversational style—not like a recited speech—in about 30 seconds or so.

This *will* require some preparation. Make a written outline if that helps. Practice it in front of a mirror. Yes, one of the exercises below will require you to rehearse it with a partner. Here is a very important point: *Do not memorize a speech!* That will sound canned and phony. Remember the basic elements of what you want to say and convey those conversationally. The single most important piece of advice here is to know yourself and be comfortable in your own skin.

HELPFUL WEBSITES

The following websites might provide you with useful information regarding job vacancies, internships, upcoming educational meetings, and other professional development opportunities:

www.ache.org—American College of Healthcare Executives

www.mgma.org—Medical Group Management Association

www.himss.org—Health Information and Management Systems Society

http://www.ahcancal.org/—American Health Care Association

www.nahse.org—National Association of Health Services Executives

www.shsmd.org—Society for Healthcare Strategy and Market Development

www.hfma.org—Healthcare Financial Management Association

www.hiaa.org—Health Insurance Association of America

www.ashrm.org—American Society for Healthcare Risk Management

CONCLUSION

In some ways, networking is something we do every day. Material in this chapter should help you think about the process a bit more clearly and develop some skills and techniques to improve the process of networking so it can be more meaningful to you. For some, these techniques are very difficult; for others, it may come more naturally. In either case, networking can and will play an important role in establishing your professional reputation. This is why we started with "Who You Are" in Chapter 1 and then moved to "The First Impression" in Chapter 2. This is the place where you can marry the concepts from those chapters to the information in this chapter and help yourself move your career ahead. Engaging in this process will help you learn *something*, and will also help you develop an acquaintanceship with *someone*. That is what networking is all about.

Observations from the Professionals

The Importance of Networking

Anthony C. Stanowski, DHA, FACHE, is the vice president for Applied Medical Software, Collingswood, NJ. He serves on the boards of Bon Secours Baltimore Health System, in Baltimore, MD, and the Commission on Accreditation of Healthcare Management Education, in Washington, DC. Anthony previously held executive positions at ARAMARK, Philadelphia (PA), Thomson Reuters Healthcare (IL), and at several Philadelphia area based providers, including Jefferson Health System. He served as President of the Healthcare Planning and Marketing Society of New Jersey.

When I was a graduate student, my professor's exhortations about networking seemed irrelevant. I felt that if I knew my material well, worked hard, and produced results, I would succeed. I had skills . . . hard technical skills . . . and a fine education pedigree. Networking, I thought, was for those who did not have the credentials, and who needed to glad-hand to get ahead.

My misguided impression of networking was of soulless scoundrels who populate association meetings pressing their business cards by handshake as they flitter from person to person. While they are talking to one person, their eyes dart around the room searching for a more important executive who can better elevate their career.

I was so wrong.

I am now going to tell you the most important thing about networking. It is a paradox. Networking is NOT about you, or getting others to do something for you. Networking is about serving others, without an expectation of return. When you do this well, you will succeed.

Networking is not quick and easy. It is not simply measured in LinkedIn network connections, or friends on Facebook. It is a lifetime process of building relationships that matter. Just as a marriage (or any significant relationship) is work, so is business networking. And like a good marriage, you should be enjoying yourself during the process.

Woody Allen said that 80% of life is just showing up. Electronic networking (blogs, LinkedIn, Facebook, etc.) are part of the tool kit, but being there in person is not to be underestimated. Communications takes many forms; utilize them all.

As a young careerist, the question is how to start? Here are five not-so-easy tips to help you begin.

1. *Make connections inside your own company or university program.* Who are you having lunch with? Are you participating on the company softball team or in the student club? Do you volunteer for community activities sponsored by your company or college? What about the blood drive? The United Way? Hospitals are incredibly social organizations, and there is always something going on. Geez . . . I still have the flashlight from when, as a young administrative fellow, I directed Philadelphia's elite to their seats at Graduate Hospital's "Fair in the Square" fundraiser.

    The importance of networking within your hospital or college is that people eventually leave that place. Being connected at your organization is the first stepping stone to build your reputation outside of your facility.

2. *Grow your network outside of your organization.* Find people who share your interests. The American College of Healthcare Executives has a strong local network that is always looking for volunteers. Are you interested in finance? Look at the local Healthcare Financial Management Association chapters. Marketing? Search for Society for Healthcare Strategy and Market Development local groups. Do you come from a diverse background? There are multiple national organizations that have many local chapters, such as the National Association of Health Services Executives. Attend local chapter meetings, and have a genuine passion for the group's work.

    If associations are not your thing, then maybe your alma mater needs you. Sure, you graduated, and maybe you still have a small grudge against that finance professor for giving you a B that messed up your perfect 4.0 average. But get over it! Participate in fund-raisers. Look, the university knows you just got out of school, but you can donate something, can't you? Are there educational events going on at campus? Volunteer to help staff them.

3. *Roll up your sleeves and make things happen.* Get involved! Sure, you are busy. Well, we all are busy! The networker is just busy getting ahead.

    Call up the *chief networker*, also known as the society president, committee chair, or alumni director. Ask where they need help and volunteer. Start small to show you are dependable: check people in, print out name badges, and call people the day before the meeting to make sure they are coming.

    Once you volunteer, complete on time and professionally what you volunteered for. Treat your work with the association just like you would treat your work in your job. Meet deadlines, provide updates, and ask for advice in completing the project. And look, everyone is busy, so do not use that as an excuse for missing your assignment.

    The reward for completing your assignments is that you are asked to do more, like chair a committee, or serve on the executive board. Most importantly, you will amass a great network that you can count on.

4. *Treat everyone with respect,* but especially these three groups:

    a. *Security guards and maintenance staff.* These are the people who are circulating every day throughout your facility and know everyone. Smile, and say hello. Learn their names. One of ARAMARK's maintenance people noticed that I did not have a lunch scheduled for a very important meeting that included several partner hospital CEOs. He searched me out, and asked me if that was correct. He saved me from a disaster.

    b. *Administrative assistants.* These are the gate-keepers to executives, but inevitably there are those who put on an aura of superiority to an assistant. This fails every time, as an assistant not just controls an executive's calendar, but also is a key confidant.

    c. *Salespeople.* Salespeople are a way to expand your network exponentially. They are the best networkers; they have to be to get their job completed! Take salespeoples' calls. First, be honest, and do not waste their time. Ask them about what other companies are doing. Can they put you in touch with their clients who are working on a project similar to yours? Are you interviewing at another hospital? Your salesperson may know the contact there, and may be able to give you some information about the company, or even recommend you.

5. *Help others succeed in their career.* If you know a colleague who suddenly has found themself out of a job, give him or her a call. Volunteer your assistance. People do not forget those who helped them at their lowest level. When you get that call from a headhunter and it is not the right position for you, suggest a friend who is out of a job, and then immediately call that person to alert them that a recruiter will call. Are there positions open at your organization that you think would be a good fit for a colleague? Let people know.

Through this process of helping others, you will develop a network that you can depend upon as you grow your career. More importantly, your career journey will be far more fulfilling because of the people you met, and helped, along the way.

EXERCISES

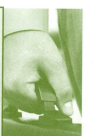

4-1. Develop an outline for an "elevator speech." Write it out if you choose, but do not memorize the speech. Remember the points you want to make. Practice with a recorder and/or in front of a mirror.

4-2. Practice your elevator speech with a partner. Time one another. Did your partner tell you (and did you tell your partner) something about your student status, your professional interests, your passion, your strengths, and how others would describe you? Be candid with each other in your assessment.

4-3. Identify someone who is an appropriate person with whom an informational interview would be interesting. Schedule to meet with that person. Prepare questions you want to ask, focusing on the health care industry, the person's organization, and their career path.

4-3. Find a partner with whom to engage in a role play. Pretend one of you is a student attending a large, national professional conference; the other is a CEO of a prestigious organization in that industry sector. You saw the CEO speak at a session earlier in the day. Start a conversation.
Reverse roles and repeat.
Evaluate one another using the information from this chapter.

BIBLIOGRAPHY

Abroms, B., Fillmore, M., & Marczinski, C. (2003). Alcohol-Induced Impairment of Behavioral Control: Effects on the Alteration and Suppression of Prepotent Responses. *Journal of Studies on Alcohol*, 687–695.

Taylor, J. (2012, March 6). *Non-Awkward Ways To Start and End Networking Conversations*. Retrieved May 15, 2012, from Forbes.com: http://www.forbes.com

White, A. (2004, July). *What Happened? Alcohol, Memory Blackouts and the Brain*. Retrieved June 4, 2012, from Natonal Institute on Alcohol Abuse and Alcoholism: http://pubs.niaaa.nih.gov/publications

Chapter 5

The Cover Letter: Get the Door Open!

There is one purpose and only one purpose of a cover letter: to persuade the recipient that you are enough of a viable candidate for the job that the employer should take the time to talk with you about the job, fellowship, residency, or internship. To do this, the letter must (a) be brief enough that the addressee will read it; (b) present an interesting enough picture of you to capture their attention; (c) have something in it that differentiates you professionally from other candidates; and, (d) lead the reader to examine your résumé. In this chapter you will learn the basic elements of a cover letter; how to develop one that casts you in the most favorable light; and the types of circumstances that might lead you to send a cover letter and how those circumstances should change the letter.

BASIC ELEMENTS

Before we get into the meat of what a letter should contain and how it should be done, there is one constant about a cover letter to address: never ever send your letter without a résumé. The letter is a significant part of the package, but not the *whole* package. While résumés are the subject of the next chapter, these two go together like hand and glove.

Before You Begin: The Stationery and the Font

Not only does the content of the cover letter need to be compelling enough for the reader to want to learn more about you, the letter needs to be eye-catching as well. This is somewhat tricky. To be clear, do not use pastel paper or paper with decorated borders. If you send a letter on light blue stationery with a fancy border around the edges . . . well, it is hard to make your point from the trash can. Unless you are applying for a position that involves demonstrating your artful creativity (In which case, why are you reading *this* book?), your letter and résumé should be on stationery paper—that is to say linen paper—available at any book store or office supply shop. The color can be light beige or light gray. Avoid the temptation to be cute: it will not help. The *image* or *brand* of you as a professional for the reader, in many cases, begins right here.

Your second decision is which font to use. Computers have made it possible to have a choice from among a wide assortment of fonts, making it wonderfully easy to be creative. But remember, aside from being distinctive, "creativity" has its limits in this context. The first choice is serif or no serif.

A font with a serif is the most widely used and recognized font in today's world. This style is a holdover from the invention of the Guttenberg press. The typesetters back then needed a way to make the letters stay mounted on a line and that little curve at the edge of the letter worked. As a consequence, most of the things we see in print today use some form of a serif font; take a look at this textbook, or any other, the local newspaper, *The New York Times*, and almost any book, including e-books. Because of the widespread prevalence of the use of fonts with serifs, we have adapted to read it more easily; it is something we are accustomed to seeing.

Whether serif or sans serif is more legible is a matter of debate. There are a number of factors that weigh on the issues of legibility and readability, such as point size and things like *x-height* and *counters*, which are well beyond the scope of this book (Poole, 2008). The point is you have a choice between the two. This is an example of that notion of style discussed in Chapter 2. At the end of the day, there is no conclusive evidence that one is "better" than the other. Many hold the belief that because we see the serif font every day we are more accustomed to seeing it and that, therefore, it is easier to read—that somehow the sans serif font contributes to eye fatigue. Conversely, *because* the serif font is used so widely, perhaps *distinctive* means you should use a sans serif font, or perhaps a different form of serif font. You will find examples of both styles below. The strong points and criticisms in the examples apply to both.

The Letterhead

There are probably thousands of ways to make a letterhead. With computers, you have it in your power to create a masterpiece. Again, however, resist the temptation to go overboard. This is one of those (many) places in life that "just because you can, does not mean you should" applies. Your letterhead should be free of clutter; have a *clean* look; be easy to read; and reflect your professionalism. The four serif samples shown here will show you two examples that look good and two that need improvement. See Figure 5-1 as a sample of what to avoid.

There are several things that need improvement here. Notice the font. The example here is a 12-point

ERIC F. GOFAR
1234 Polo Court ♦ Columbia, Missouri 69812 ♦ 843.708.8636
gofar@stateu.edu

Figure 5–1 A letterhead example with a small font and cluttered style.

font called Cambria. It is closely related to Times New Roman, perhaps a small—almost unnoticeable—bit larger. The name, however, should be slightly larger than the contact information, perhaps 14- or 16-point size. Consider, however, if this were the Constantina font—which is noticeably larger than Times New Roman—then you would want to reconsider both the size of the name and the size of the font throughout the document. The other point about this particular example is that the name is in all caps. Again, because of the way we are accustomed to reading, using all caps makes this a bit more challenging to the eye. Yes, the name can (and should) be somewhat distinctive. But not in a way that strains the eye of the reader. Finally, note the second line of the letterhead. By placing the phone number so close to the zip code, the string of numbers resembles a bank account. Avoid this look for the same reason: the reader needs to slow down to ferret out the phone number from all that information. In my other example of what to avoid, see Figure 5-2.

The text in Figure 5-2 is a bit better, but still not quite the look one should have for a letterhead. Note that the zip code and phone number are in different places, which is a good start. Here the problem

Larry John Gerald
900 Jeremiah Daniel Dr. Apt. 6601 • Topeka, KS 65432
geraldl@state.edu • 555.123.6127

Figure 5–2 Another example of what to avoid; make sure your name is not too large.

is basically the size of the name. The most common thing students do in this part of the process is oversize the name. This error is not quite as egregious as some, but still the point size here is too large. Too many times students seem to think they need their names in 18- or 20-point font in order to be seen. No! Keep things within "reach" of each other. If you put your name in 18-point font and then, because your letter is a bit too long, you use an 11-point font for the body of the letter, it will look like you think you are the health administration equivalent of one of *The Avengers*. Most places are not in the market for a superhero.

As a frame of reference, if you use a 12-point Times New Roman font for your letter, your name should appear no larger than 16-point size in that same font. Ironically, the example here (Figure 5-2) is, in fact, a 16-point size. It is, however, the opposite problem we saw in the previous example. This is Palatino, which is a slightly larger font than Times New Roman and thus this name comes on just a bit strong, even if still in proportion to the rest of the text. It just seems a bit large. Now to turn to a more positive example, see Figure 5-3.

In Figure 5-3 you can see how the letterhead is shifted over to the left and the author used a line to separate her name from the contact information. This is about as artistic as you should get. She used a Times New Roman font and kept things in proportion by using a 14-point font for her name and 12-point font for the contact information. Notice the other thing she did here that has a good look—she put her name in bold, which makes for a nice contrast to the rest of the letter. This letterhead has just enough of an artist's touch to be attractive and somewhat distinctive. Figure 5-4 shows the more traditional look.

Alexandra Campbell Fails
1234 New Vista Terrace
Kansas City, MO 62166
Telephone: (555) 771-8989
Email: fails@state.edu

Figure 5–4 An example of a "traditional" letterhead style.

This is a classic look, featuring a nice-sized serif font. The name is appropriately proportioned to the rest of the text. It has a *clean* look; everything is in order and appears where it should logically be. While not particularly distinctive in an artful way, this is *tried and true* in that it is the classic, conservative look for a letterhead. You will not be penalized by the reader for using this format.

Now look at Figures 5-5 and 5-6. Figure 5-5 is in Arial, which seems like the sans serif equivalent to Palatino—it still seems just a bit large. Figure 5-6 is in Calibri and still looks appropriately sized. You should try several variations to find a style that you believe reflects who you are. Once you have settled on that, use the same configuration—the same font,

---

Larry John Gerald
900 Jeremiah Daniel Dr. Apt. 6601 • Topeka, KS 65432
geraldl@state.edu • 555.123.6127

Figure 5–5 Letterhead using Arial font.

Joanie Sharpknife
5512 Cutem Rd., #666
Scalpel, SC 29412
(863) 555-6789
sharpknife@gmail.com

Figure 5–3 An example of a good, clean letterhead style.

Joanie Sharpknife
5512 Cutem Rd., #666
Scalpel, SC 29412
(863) 555-6789
sharpknife@gmail.com

Figure 5–6 Try several fonts and sizes to see which suits you best. Calibri is used here.

the same sizes, the same layout for the header of your résumé. More on that in Chapter 6, but for now, as you think about this choice, think about how it will look on your résumé as well.

One final thought about fonts. The body of the letter and the letterhead should be in identical fonts. While some would argue that being in the same family of fonts is sufficient, for your purposes keep it simple by avoiding those artistic questions and stay focused on what works best for accomplishing the goal of getting your message across. Use one font.

THE BODY OF THE LETTER: MAKE *THE PITCH* IN ONE PAGE

Now that you have the right look and feel in terms of stationery and font, you need to craft a letter that will invite the reader—perhaps even compel the reader—to invite you for an interview. The letter is an important document. What you say here, and how you say it, can make the difference in "getting in the door."

Getting Noticed

Some people are not comfortable with calling attention to themselves for reasons best known to them; however, you can gain some attention right off the top by how you structure the inside address of the letter. Figure 5-7 is a good example of how you can make your letter distinctive quickly and easily.

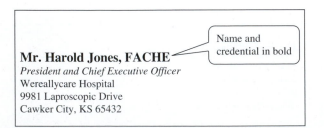

Figure 5–7 Try putting the recipient's name and credentials in bold for an eye-catching look.

Note the recipient's name is in bold and the title is in italics. This has a terrific look; it expresses the importance of the recipient and his role. Pay particular attention to the use of the credential *FACHE* after the name. Always include the credential(s) the person has attained, if you are aware of his achievements. It shows good attention to detail. In addition, the recipient has gone to a lot of work to get that extra degree or certification and will appreciate the acknowledgment. This example also includes "Mr." This is optional. When addressing a woman, the modern convention is "Ms." When addressing a medical doctor or doctor of philosophy, either one of two ways is appropriate. "Dr. Tom Jones" is fine; so is "Tom Jones, MD" or "Tom Jones, PhD." If the recipient has achieved some additional distinction, like the FACHE credential, and is also a doctor of one kind or the other, then consider using "Dr. Tom Jones, FACHE," though "Tom Jones, PhD, FACHE" is also acceptable. The academic achievement is sufficiently advanced that it deserves treatment separate from an additional professional certification. Thus, it should always precede the professional credential. To reiterate the point from earlier in the book: a female PhD or MD is no less a "doctor" than a male who has the same degree. If you make the mistake of addressing a female who has this advanced degree as "Ms." or "Mrs." without noting the degree after her name, you likely will not be considered. Young men have made this mistake countless times and it implicitly devalues the woman recipient and her accomplishment. Do not make this mistake.

Making the Pitch

Your cover letter should be no more than three or four paragraphs long. Unless there are special circumstances (to be addressed later in this chapter), it generally should be only a one page, especially for something like an undergraduate internship. For a graduate fellowship, it *may* be appropriate to go to a second page. Be cautious about this and do it only if really necessary. Keep in mind that the reader is busy. She has not been sitting around playing Angry Birds waiting for your letter to arrive. Depending on the position for which you are applying, there may be 100—or more—applicants, all of whom believe they will be the future CEO. Keep it brief. You are not writing your autobiography. You are, however, introducing yourself briefly and, just as briefly, making a case for why you are a "fit" for the position in question.

A good cover letter, as we can see in Figure 5-8, will have three elements.

The Opening

In the opening paragraph of the letter you need to establish three things. First, introduce yourself; second, explain how you know of them or their organization; and third, tell the reader what you want from them. That is it. Do not start with "my name is." They know your name from the letterhead and the signature block. Repeating it here will sound like fingernails scratching a chalkboard.

The Pitch

This is the second paragraph and represents the heart of the letter. The single most important message here—whether this is an undergrad internship, a graduate fellowship, or a routine job—is you telling the reader what you can do for their organization. Plenty of times students will talk about "This is the experience I need to help my career" or words to that effect. Be cognizant of the fact, from the reader's perspective, it really *is not* about you. This is where you talk about the results you have had in the past as an example of what *you* can do for *them*. Talk about your education—specific projects that demonstrate skills you can put to work for *them*. In some cases, you may want to use bullets to list a few things or even move to a columnar format.

The Close

Ask for an interview; mention how you will follow up. The best practice is for you to keep the initiative and mention that you will call their office within a reasonable period of time, like 10 days or two weeks, to see if a time can be arranged that is mutually convenient. This may seem forward, but it also shows seriousness and desire on your part. One thing employers everywhere are looking for is employees who are self-starters; who can complete projects; and, who can work well with others and be an impactful leader. You can never be an impactful leader without being at least mildly assertive on occasion. In our example, the writer handled it exactly right; she pointed out her contact information in the event the reader wanted to call her, but she retained the "I want to do this" posture by saying if she did not hear from them that she would call.

When to Use a Cover Letter

Figure 5-8 provides a good example of the kind of letter one should use, but it is *not a one size fits all* proposition. Clearly, the letter reveals that the organization does, in fact, have an established summer internship program. The writer is applying to a known entity; an existing program. It is also obvious that it comes from a student who is motivated and focused on an internship experience. The language tells us that. So while it makes a good template, this is where you should apply what you have learned about yourself from Chapter 1. Are you willing "to take on any task" and have a "sense of pride" in your work? You cannot—well, should not—just "lift" the language here and apply it in your own letter. Taking the language and using it as your own would be unethical—and that will be addressed later in the book. But not only would it be an act of plagiarism to take the language, it would not reflect who *you* are—which is what the employer really wants to know. Frankly, if you got a job under some kind of pretense being someone else, what fun would that be for you when you discover you do not fit in very well? So, use the template, the format, but not the language.

This is an important concept, because there are several other circumstances in which you would write a cover letter. Thus, in addition to our example of an undergraduate (or MHA) internship, you will need to adapt the language—that is, *your* language—to other contexts. The times that you will need a cover letter are

1. applying for a residency or fellowship;
2. applying for an advertised job vacancy;
3. following up on a networking lead; and
4. perhaps a "cold call" to an executive.

Joanie Sharpknife

5512 Cutem Rd., #666

Scalpel, SC 29412

(863) 555-6789

sharpknife@gmail.com

September 20, 2011

> Very nice introductory paragraph; explains self; how she knew of this opportunity; level of interest is clear.

Ms. Catherine Cutyourself, FACHE
President and Chief Executive Officer
Slicem & Dicem Hospital
Waynesboro, USA 23456

Dear Ms. Cutyourself:

Please consider this letter and accompanying resume my application for a summer internship at Sicem & Dicem Hospital. I learned of your program through students and faculty who spoke very highly of your organization. Originally from Mission Hills, KS, I had the opporrunity to attend Washington University, in St. Louis, MO, for my undergraduate studies and moved to Collegetown, PA to complete a Master in Health Administration at the University of Allknowing. Throughout college I had a wide variety of interests. Because I spent a great deal of time around the health care system, I developed an interest in healthcare administration. As a result, I majored in Business Administration with the intention of pursuing a graduate degree in Healthcare Administration.

I am in the process of completing my first year in Allknowing's MHA Program. This knowledge I am developing will be a great foundation for a summer work experience in your hospital. My past work history is very good. Former employers would tell you that I am energetic, helpful and eager to learn. While I do not yet have any significant healthcare management experience, several of the skills I learned elsewhere will transfer to the health care setting. For example, in my summer job last year I created a pro forma demonstrating the value in purchasing a new piece of equipment. Additionally, I was a member of a team in a national case competition focused on issues of patient safety and systems-based practice.

> Acknowledges lack of experience, but speaks to education, a successful project, and a relevant co-curricular activity

Because of my sense of pride in my work and willingness to take on any task, I look forward to learning more about your organization and to sharing more about myself. I can be reached at the contact information provided above; however, I will follow up by contacting your office in the next two weeks.

> Good closing; mentions work ethic; indicates she will call if she doesn't hear from them first

Sincerely,

Joanie Sharpknife

Figure 5–8 A good cover letter will have three elements: the introduction, the pitch, and the close.

Applying for Residency or Fellowship

MHA students applying for a residency or fellowship, or undergrads looking for a summer internship, can use a letter that looks a lot like the one in Figure 5-8. Indeed, if you are a first year (MHA) student, you can use seeking the internship as practice for the residency or fellowship application process. But, of course, it should not be an identical letter.

Whenever possible, at this level and beyond, you will want to tailor the letter to the stated requirements for the residency or fellowship. Sometimes this means you may want to refer to the organization's Mission Statement in the letter. Other times you may include something the organization has done recently that was noteworthy in some way. Likewise, you *will* want to integrate some recent experience from your program—either curricular or co-curricular—that demonstrates competencies in the area of interpersonal skills, communication, or successful execution of a project. It is doubtful you can get all three in a one-page letter, but at this level it may be more important to be fully expressive than to artificially limit yourself to one page.

In this residency or fellowship process, generally, organizations are seeking people (1) of good character; (2) who are highly talented; (3) who present themselves professionally; (4) who demonstrate the ability to work well with others; (5) who demonstrate critical thinking/problem solving skills; and (6) who can communicate clearly and appropriately with people from all levels in the organization. Thus, your cover letter, combined with your résumé, need to provide enough insight about you to demonstrate you have the ability to meet these requirements.

Applying for an Advertised Job Vacancy

Here is where the cover letter really needs to be tailor made for the recipient. They have given you some terrific material to use in the form of the advertisement or the posting. Look carefully at the qualifications they seek. Apart from the degrees, what skills or competencies are mentioned in the ad that fit your particular skill set? See Figure 5-9 for an excellent example of how to respond to this situation.

Note that this letter has followed all the guidelines discussed above: clean, easy-to-read letterhead; proportional sizing of name to text; consistent use of font; and bold and italics in the inside address. From a technical perspective, the letter is perfect.

Now take a look at the column of comparisons. Note that the requirements and qualifications match up beautifully. Even more importantly, notice how the references in the "My Experience" column are very specific. Not only has the writer used MapPoint, but tells how—and this reference is doubly important because this is the kind of study (distribution of cardiac surgery volumes) that would be critically important in a planning department, which is the subject of the posted advertisement. Each of those references is specific to the announced job qualification and done in a specific way to underscore the value of this gentleman's experience as being relevant to what the organization seeks in this position.

Following Up on a Networking Lead

As you saw in the last chapter, networking is a critically important skill to have in not only looking for a job, but in developing a position of strength in the profession; having a wide variety of friends and acquaintances upon whom you can call for referrals, information, or just someone to commiserate with. But if you are in job searching mode, then this becomes all the more important. Likewise, the follow up with those contacts is magnified even more.

This section is not about those people on whom you have called for an "informational" interview to whom you send a thank you note—that was covered in the last chapter. This section is about following up on more casual leads that you may uncover at a national, regional, or local professional meeting. This letter needs to be an outgrowth of the conversation that has led you to writing. Thus, while the template may be similar, introduce, pitch, and close, the wording will be unique to reflect the circumstances.

Therefore, for example, the *introductory* paragraph becomes more of a *reminder*, as in, "It was a real pleasure to meet you last week at the MGMA annual meeting. I enjoyed our conversation about the

Robert Luke Franks
1213 Cameron Way
Tempe, AZ 85012
(555) 345-9876
rlfranks@provider.com

December 15, 2012

Mr. Christopher Jonathan
Chief Operating Officer
The Wellbe Healthcare System
9901 Hospital Drive
Colorado Springs, CO   76543

Dear Mr. Jonathan:

The Wellbe Healthcare System (WHS) has a reputation all across the Western US that has captured my attention and earned my respect. That you are now seeking a Senior Planning Analyst affords me the opportunity to join your organization. Please consider this letter and accompanying resume my application.

   A careful review of my qualifications and the requirements included in the advertisement in this month's edition of *Healthcare Executive*, suggests I am well qualified for this important position.

Your Requirements	My Experience
• Ability to work with Microsoft MapPoint	• Used MapPoint to display cardiac surgery volumes for the entire state in my MHA Capstone Project
• Advanced quantitative skills	• Used SPSS to analyze relationship of cardiac volumes to quality of care
• Excellent oral and written communication skills	• National champion in Clarion Case Competition (2010)
	• 2d place – ACHE Essay Competition (2011)
• Demonstrated ability to work in team environment	• Led team effort to produce in depth market analysis of helipad and trauma service in major metro area

As I complete my Administrative Fellowship at St. Xavier's, I am looking for an opportunity to make a valuable contribution to an organization such as WHS. My resume is enclosed for your convenience. I will call next week to request an appointment, or you may reach me at the contact information above. Thank you for your time and consideration.

Sincerely,

Robert L. Franks

Enclosure

Figure 5–9 An example of a cover letter responding to an advertised job vacancy.

growth in ambulatory surgery volumes." No one can give you boilerplate language to fit every situation; you need to make the association in the letter strong enough so that the reader will remember.

And the second paragraph may be both a *reminder* and a *pitch* as in, "You mentioned that your Denver office may be looking for a new executive director, a position for which my education and experiences make me well suited. I am following up on our conversation because I believe I could make a positive contribution in the circumstances you described." Same concept as before: what can you do for them?

Finally, the close can be quite similar. Make a point of calling attention to the résumé you have enclosed. Refer to your contact information if they want to reach you; but note that you will follow up in the next week or 10 days.

Of course, most of these conversations will not be about specific positions. Life just is not that easy! Most often these conversations will be as follows: "We're building a new bed tower and I know at some point we will need some additional people to help oversee the facilities function." Or it might be "We don't have anything right now, but a friend of mine at Wellbe Health System said they are looking for a new planning analyst." So the letter you write will need to be tailored to fit that situation. Here, in the first case you might make a reference to the conversation and provide your information so that as they get closer to assessing their needs, you might be interested in talking with them. Again, follow up. This time, do follow up, but in a timeframe that seems reasonable in the context of the conversation. That could be one week or two months. It is a judgment call that needs to fit the urgency—or lack of it—in the need expressed. If the bed tower is nearly complete, then to follow up sooner compared to the bed tower that is just breaking ground would make some sense. Likewise, in the case "I heard there may be something at Wellbe," your letter should inquire if the reader would mind either sharing your information with his friend or if he would permit you to use his name when you contact his friend. In today's world, you might cover all this via e-mail as opposed to snail mail.

The Cold Call Cover Letter

One may question the value of even doing this, because most of the time this letter will end up in the trash. But, it is included here because it is still possible that someone will read it and respond affirmatively. This letter can look like either of our two examples (Figure 5-8 and Figure 5-9); however, again the context requires a change in the language. It is a bit of a disadvantage: you do not know the recipient and there is no advertised job with criteria listed against which to compare your experience. Nonetheless, if you are moving to a city where you do not know anyone, this may be a strategy you undertake for at least a little while.

In cases like this, the letter needs to be slightly more generic. If you have done some research on the organization to which you are writing (recommended), you can mention your interest in using your skills to support whatever initiative it is that caught your interest. The introduction and pitch paragraphs will be more generic. They, nonetheless, should reflect your skills, your interests, and how you can affect a positive outcome at whatever organization it may be. Then close the letter referenced previously: provide your contact information, but be certain to mention that you will be in touch "in the near future," probably 10 days to two weeks.

SOME THINGS TO AVOID

A fair amount of material about *writing* was covered in Chapter 2. Because we are talking about a specific type of correspondence in this chapter, we will be a bit more specific here.

1. Do not use contractions. Do not use "I'm"—it is "I am."
2. Do not abbreviate the first reference to a word. For example, "gastroenterology" becomes "GI" only after you have introduced the initials in ( ) following the first use of the word.
3. Avoid fragments and run-on sentences. Finish the thought in the former; consider breaking the latter into two sentences.

A FEW WORDS ABOUT ELECTRONIC APPLICATIONS

Sometimes all of this formatting and making things look "just so" will be for naught as the prospective employer will require submission of materials in an electronic format. This can take place in several ways so be aware.

First, and most direct, is requiring applicants to e-mail documents to apply for a position. In this case, you should still go through all the steps we discussed in this chapter and in Chapter 6 that follows with respect to formatting the letter and the résumé. While you do not need to be concerned with stationery, the formatting will still be important to the appearance of the document. To assure the formatting remains intact after transmittal, convert your documents from whatever word processing program you have used to create them to a PDF format. That will keep your margins and spacing lined up where you intended them to be.

Second, some employers will have a combination of "fill in the field" and "upload" technology. In this case, you should take special precaution to assure you are entering information in the fields correctly, of course. When asked to upload documents, double check the formatting requirement. If you can, upload a PDF so you can assure the best presentation of yourself. If not, then upload your document in whatever word processing format you have used, understanding that the receiving program will likely convert it to a format the employer finds convenient. At least you will be on equal footing as this will happen to all the other applicants as well. Be certain to double—triple—check all the information you have entered before hitting the final "submit" button. Accuracy is everything.

Third, some large employers will have "smart" technology that will ask you to upload your documents and will then auto-fill fields of information with data taken from your résumé. You probably will need to make some corrections, so, again, review the information with great care to assure its accuracy. This same system will also ask you to upload your letter and/or personal statement as well so your entire application will be in electronic format for the employer's review.

The use of electronic applications has grown significantly in recent years. As systems have become perfected and more sophisticated, employers have become more comfortable with their use. Because of that, the use of this technology is expanding, so we will see more electronic applications in the future, particularly for entry level positions, expanding to mid-level positions over time.

THE USE AND ABUSE OF E-MAIL

The advent of e-mail has exponentially expanded the amount of "information" any of us receive. If you are writing to a busy executive, consider that he or she may be receiving 100, 200, or more, e-mails per day. For the sake of argument, let us say she receives 90. Now imagine spending, on average, one minute per e-mail. There goes one and one-half hours of her day. Sure, some get trashed before they are opened, but some will take several minutes. The point here is if you e-mail someone—anyone, really—for any reason, be respectful of that person's time.

Be clear in what you say in an e-mail; be particularly careful because if there is a chance what you say can be misinterpreted, chances are good it will. Use a clear, brief subject line. Write in crisp, brief sentences.

Keep it short. If you write more than five sentences, use the first sentence to explain the reason for writing. Consider writing a memo and attaching it to the e-mail; then use the subject line to say, for example "New CT; negative recommendation; one page memo attached." This way the reader knows what is going on before opening the e-mail. The reader can read the memo when it is convenient to him. (*Note:* Try to be brief when writing memos. Keeping them to one page is best.)

Consider using the phone. If an issue requires resolution through give and take, the sharing of ideas and perspectives, back and forth, use e-mail to schedule a telephone conversation or "teleconference." If you get in this game of electronic table tennis of going back and forth via e-mail, it really increases the chances for a misunderstanding. Your job—always—is to facilitate communication and make it easier for information to flow where it needs to be in a timely fashion. If something requires a discussion to make that happen, then have a real discussion, not a collection of one-way pixelated flotsam.

Avoid fancy fonts, background colors, graphics as signatures, colorful borders, and pastel backgrounds. All of that (a) distracts from the message and (b) takes more time to open.

When you are passing along information, especially if you are passing it to someone higher in the organization, do not merely forward the entire thread and say "See the conversation below." If you send this to a VP he will wonder what good you are. If it is necessary to provide the thread so the reader can find the detail if they choose, fine. Your note should be a summary of the decision, the information, or whatever the topic is. Add value to the communication by clarifying the matter and reducing it to its most basic elements.

Do not cc the entire western world unless it is really necessary. The only people who need to see the copies are those directly associated with the conversation or project. It is particularly poor form to cc someone else's boss. How would *you* feel if someone did that to you? Using cc in this way is really a way of whining to someone about something you think is not fair, appropriate, or necessary. Do not. If you have that

kind of issue, then address it professionally with the person you believe is the source of your angst. Do it in person. Do not include others in this kind of discussion unless necessary and central to the issue you are raising.

When replying, do not use the *reply all* button unless it is absolutely necessary. Let us say someone is trying to schedule a meeting with 10 people for next Wednesday at 2 PM and you are one of the 10. You *reply all* that the time and date are fine with you; you have just put nine e-mails in boxes of people who really do not need to know if you are available. Assume it takes 30 seconds to open, read, and discard the e-mail. The total (wasted) time consumed is 4.5 minutes. If everyone in this meeting did that, then there would be 81 unnecessary e-mails. At 30 seconds each, that is 40.5 minutes of productive time wasted. And if there were six of those kinds of meetings and similar responses (and there are a *lot* of meetings, especially in hospitals), that is approximately 4.3 hours of time wasted. Do not be the person who contributes to this. The only person who needs to know is the organizer. Send your reply to him or her and no one else.

Do not use e-mail to vent frustration or complain or attack someone or something. This is an invitation to an electronic squabble that could escalate beyond all reason. Again, if you have that kind of frustration, take it up directly with the person involved. Control the impulse to spout off. It will only make matters worse.

When asking how you can help, be specific? Do not ask "Thoughts?" or "How can I help?" Be specific. Offer options to the recipient. "Can I help by (a) completing the project myself; (b) offering to support Roger in getting it done; or, (c) staying out of it?" This is brief and to the point and provides the recipient to be brief in response.

The rule of thumb is, generally, be brief and be respectful of other people's time. E-mail is a valuable tool for many, many things. Abusing it by being verbose or using it inappropriately, however, results in misunderstanding and a waste of time.

CONCLUSION

The letter has three parts: the introduction; the pitch; and the close. It generally should be one page, though sometimes there are circumstances where a second page could be appropriate. Tailor the letter as specifically as possible to the circumstances; the letter is the invitation to review your résumé. Together, those are the ticket that gets you in the door. Finally, write effectively, using appropriate language that describes you and your skills. Of course, do not forget to tell the reader the kind of value you can bring to their organization. Finally, always, always include your résumé.

Observations from the Professionals

What We Look for in a Personal Statement

Jeffery Knorr is administrative director for Women's Health Services for the University of Pittsburgh Medical Center (UPMC) physician practices. UPMC is a 22-hospital integrated health care system in Western Pennsylvania that includes 2,700 physicians representing virtually all medical specialties. UPMC is the academic health system for the University of Pittsburgh medical school and its flagship hospital is ranked 10th nationally by U.S. News and World Report.

Like the professional résumé, the value of the personal statement is often assessed by the individual preference of the reader. Attempting to understand how individual preferences are formed for one style of personal statement over another would be an exercise in futility. However, as someone who has written many personal statements, both as an undergraduate and graduate health care administration student at Penn State, and as someone who has reviewed hundreds as a member of the Administrative Fellowship recruitment committee at the University of Pittsburgh Medical Center, I feel that I am well positioned to outline the key components of effective personal statements.

Personal statements are commonly requested by recruitment committees to be used as a crucial component of the screening process. As an applicant, your priority must be to provide your reader with a positive, last impression of who you are as a person and aspiring health care professional. Think of the screening process as a stack of applications being sorted into two piles: accepted and rejected. That might seem harsh or overly simplified, but that is the reality. You may have superior interviewing skills, but your application package will dictate whether or not you get the chance to sit at the table. When drafting your personal statement, the critical question that you must ask yourself is, "How am I positively differentiating myself from other applicants?" In my opinion, all great personal statements have the following four characteristics in common: they should be personal, professional, focused and sincere.

PERSONAL

This may seem implied, but your personal statement should actually be *personal*. If it reads like a continuation of your cover letter or résumé you have not satisfied the assignment. The reader should learn something about you that they would not otherwise be able to ascertain. This is your opportunity to provide a unique insight into who you are and what makes you the candidate that the committee simply cannot overlook. In the exceedingly competitive health care workplace, the personal statement may be your greatest opportunity to differentiate yourself from other applicants.

Tip: Write about something that is truly important to you. The personal touch will come naturally and will help your message resonate with your reader.

PROFESSIONAL

A common misconception is that establishing a personal connection results in a sacrifice of professionalism. I would argue that the most effective personal statements seamlessly integrate both elements. A professional tone can be conveyed through your word choices, formatting, and attention to detail. A thoughtful, professional approach to writing is a nice complement to a personal message.

Tip: Choose a traditional font (you cannot go wrong with Times New Roman). Also, you should format your personal statement in the same manner as your résumé and cover letter (headers, footers, page numbers, etc.).

FOCUSED

Your personal statement should be written with one specific "take-away" in mind. If you attempt to convey too many unique messages you will likely diminish the value of your desired "take-away." I would suggest creating an outline that builds entirely from one specific message that you want the reader to distinguish.

Tip: Have a colleague proofread your drafts. If they cannot easily grasp your "take-away" message you know you have some work to do.

SINCERE AND HONEST

As previously stated, your personal statement should leave a positive, lasting impression on your reader. In order to achieve this crucial lasting impression, you must create a connection with the reader. In my experience, sincerity can easily be felt in your writing. If the recruitment committee has doubts about the validity of your story or message, you better hope you have a strong résumé; otherwise, you are likely to squander your hopes at an interview.

Tip: Be true to your message. Exaggerating details or stretching the truth can put your integrity in doubt.

Now that we have outlined the fundamental traits of an effective personal statement, I feel it is imperative to identify some common themes among ineffective personal statements. The reality is that an ineffective personal statement has the ability to speak much louder than an exceptional one. As inherently obvious as some of these common mistakes may seem, when the pressure is on and the stakes are high you would be surprised at how easy it is to commit one or more of these costly errors.

THE "CANNED" RESPONSE

I know what you are thinking: *I will draft one personal statement, change a few names here and there, use it for all desired positions, and voila!* While this is tempting, having read scores of personal statements I can tell you that this writing shortcut is often easily detected. If perceived, you will come off as disingenuous and unwilling to give the effort necessary to complete the task with integrity. My advice would be to avoid the canned approach altogether. If you still plan to use a canned personal statement when applying to multiple institutions, for goodness sake, *please* be sure to include the correct institution name for the position. Few things will take you out of consideration faster than referring to the Mayo Clinic as Kaiser Permanente. If you take the time to tailor each of your personal statements to the specific organization I promise you it will be apparent to the recruitment committee, as well as greatly appreciated.

AMBIGUOUS CONNECTIONS

A common and often effective theme of the personal statement is telling the story of "how I got here." This approach can provide for an entertaining and informative reading experience. However, this can easily go awry if you attempt to convince the reader that two or more seemingly unrelated events or experiences have led you to where you are now. For instance, your reader is going to have a difficult time buying-in to the idea that your passion for water skiing is what led you to health care administration. Water skiing may have taught you a lot about perseverance and hard work, but did it really make you passionate about patient quality and safety? Your credibility will be damaged if your reader begins to question your rationale. If the truth is that you fell into health care administration head first because your roommate was enrolled in the major, I suggest you tell a different story!

EXCESSIVE STYLE

Your personal statement should not read like a Shakespearean sonnet. Your reader should move across your words effortlessly. The committee members are not likely to read your personal statement twice. If they feel compelled to reread it, then your message was not received. Bottom line: keep it simple.

GRAMMAR AND SPELLING

Your personal statement must be completely free of grammar and spelling errors. In the era of advanced word processing technology there is little excuse—and little tolerance—for careless mistakes. However, do not allow yourself to use this technology as a crutch. I once submitted a personal statement that included the word *imitative* in place of *initiative*. Spell check did not catch it and it was not flagged because it was still a grammatically sound sentence. *Imitative* had absolutely no context in the sentence, so guess what— I did not get the interview! Thus, I cannot stress enough the importance of diligent proofreading.

Once you have completed your first draft, can you say with confidence that you have crafted a document that will propel you forward in the interview process? If not, it may be time to revisit your message. Go beyond the ordinary themes and ideas that are on the surface, and hone on in on a message that you are truly passionate about—the rest will come easy.

EXERCISES

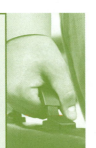

5-1. Experiment with fonts on your computer. Compare Arial to Palatino and Cambria to Times New Roman. You should type examples of 12, 14, 16, and 18 point fonts in each of them. Notice the difference? Try some other serif and sans serif combinations. Which font do you believe best suits you in the context of how you are going to use it?

5-2. Using the font you have chosen in Exercise 5-1, create a letterhead. Use any of the examples in this text, or create a new look all your own. Exchange your letterhead with a partner. Give each other constructive feedback based on the suggestions in this text.

5-3. Draft a cover letter that would be appropriate to use in applying for whatever the next step you may be taking in your education or career (Undergrad internship; MHA internship; MHA Fellowship or Residency; first job—either from undergrad or MHA program; first job after completing MHA Fellowship or Residency). Exchange your draft with a partner. Each of you should critique, carefully providing constructive feedback. Does your letter meet the guidelines suggested in this chapter?

BIIBLIOGRAPHY

Poole, A. (2008, February 17). *Which Are More Legible: Serif or Sans Serif Typefaces.* Retrieved May 17, 2012, from Alexpoole.info: http://www.alexpoole.info

Chapter 6

The Résumé: A Snapshot of Your Life

Your résumé is your introduction to others; it gives them a summary picture of who you are and, perhaps more importantly, *what* you have done. Combined with your cover letter, the résumé can help you open the door that leads to an interview. To achieve that purpose, your résumé must have a *clean* look with no extraneous matter on it; it must be detailed enough to give the reader a good idea of your skills, but not so much that it drones on and on like an autobiography. It must be a summary, but not so brief that the reader cannot get a view of your skills and accomplishments. Above all, it must be designed in a way that makes it easy for the reader to focus on the most important material.

At the end of this chapter, the student will be able to assemble a professional-looking résumé and will have an understanding of why the elements are listed in the order in which they appear. The student will also understand the importance of using action verbs to describe their accomplishments and will have an appreciation for the appropriate level of detail to include in their résumé.

THE PAPER, THE FONT, AND THE RÉSUMÉ HEAD

If you skipped over this part of Chapter 5, now would be a good time to go back and absorb that information. If you did not skip over it, now would

be a good time to return for a quick review. There is one point to make here. The paper, the font, and the "résumé" head design should be identical to that which you use for the cover letter and vice versa. ("Résumé" head is *not* a real term. The point here is that the contact information at the top of the résumé should be identical to the letterhead format). This gives a professional, no-nonsense look. Do not be tempted to get cutesy with the résumé in the belief that it needs an extra something to make certain the reader sees it. If you use pastel paper and some kind of fluffy border, the reader will see it—watching it go straight to the recycling container. Keep it simple. The cover letter and résumé should have the same stationery, font, and letterhead. Period. No exceptions.

HOW LONG SHOULD MY RÉSUMÉ BE?

There is no one magic bullet answer for this question. An academic *curriculum vitae* can be dozens of pages long, for example. In that profession, it is important to document the writer's each and every contribution to the expansion or dissemination of knowledge in their field. Thus, every publication, every presentation, and every grant are all included in the *CV*, as it is called.

The standard is quite different outside the academic world, including health care administration. The standard will also be different based on your experience, both practical and academic. Some veteran administrators with experience in the C-suite may have résumés that are six or eight pages long. At that stage of a career, it becomes a matter of style and choice, really. Some experts would say—even at that level—that those résumés are too long. Others think when you are working at that very high level, presenting a more complete picture of the candidate is appropriate.

At this stage of your career, your choices are more limited. Undergraduate résumés should seldom exceed one page. The rationale for this is straight forward: You are competing, generally, not with dozens, but with hundreds of other people for the same job. Your résumé needs to be easy to read. The recruiter is looking for one or two very specific things and needs to find them on your résumé quickly. Her review of all the résumés is going to be cursory because there are so many to be reviewed. Thus, at the undergraduate level, one page is the most beneficial length for the student. Anything longer is likely to be trashed without review.

At the master's level, the thinking is somewhat different. Generally, the pool of competition is much smaller, fewer than 100 if you are applying for a residency or fellowship. At this level you need to demonstrate mastery (it *is*, after all, a *master's* degree) in the profession. To do this, you will need to document work and academic-related experiences and do so in a way that communicates appropriate knowledge, skills, and abilities that are of interest to the employer. For that reason, at this level, a two-page résumé is closer to the norm, assuming you have indeed acquired additional experiences through internships and volunteer service to document on the résumé. If you are just adding courses, your résumé should not be any longer than one page. For the older, more experienced master's student, three pages *could* be appropriate, but for most two pages work. Granted a three-page résumé will not likely be discarded just because of its length, like the two-page résumé of an undergraduate, but this length should be the exception and not the rule.

WHAT DO I INCLUDE?

Everything that is relevant should be included on your resume. Regardless of your academic level, you should have a good summary of your academic and work achievements on your résumé. This begins at college. Your adolescence is of interest to no one but you and your parents, and perhaps the juvenile court if you were that kind of kid. When you worked as a produce stock person for a grocery store during the summer between your freshman and sophomore years, you should include that even if you think it is not relevant. It is. This shows that you are industrious; demonstrates to the reader that you shared in the financial investment in your education; and shows that you have what it takes to get up and get to a job on time, etc. The same applies for the part-time job you had waiting tables at a restaurant while you were attending college. This, too, demonstrates work ethic. It also demonstrates something about time management, as you were balancing work and academic requirements. In this case, it also shows an ability to work with people. You truly understand what it means to serve and that is a good characteristic to have and to share with others, especially potential employers. You may also have learned you hate waiting tables and are motivated, therefore, to move ahead professionally. This, too, is a good lesson: Self-awareness is an excellent attribute to possess.

It may help to think of it this way: from the employer's point of view, what is going to make the difference in getting me to the next phase of the process? Answer: things that differentiate you from other people. So the things to include are professional experience (if any), other work experience, education and relevant certification, community service activities, professional affiliations, awards, honors, leadership roles and any presentations or publications. (*Presentation* here does not mean the power point presentation you did in class.)

Even if you think the experience does not amount to much, do not sell yourself short. Include it in your résumé because it likely says much more about you than you think.

ARE THERE SOME THINGS THAT SHOULD NOT BE INCLUDED?

While it is critical to include your academic and work accomplishments, sometimes people have a temptation to include impertinent things because they think their résumé is not long enough, or has too much white space, or they just feel the need to add some things to make it look stronger. Avoid this temptation and avoid using any of the elements discussed below.

Private Matters, Personal Information, and Physical Characteristics

There are things in life that people who make hiring decisions either do not need to know, do not care to know or are barred by law from asking. Private matters that need not—and should not—be included on your résumé include your age; marital status; religious convictions; political affiliation; and sexual orientation. These have no value in terms of demonstrating your knowledge, skills, and abilities and therefore have no place in your résumé. There is one nominal exception: If you have held a leadership position in a religious-related organization, for example, where you have documented accomplishments, then that may be included. The same applies to political organizations. No one needs to know you were a member of college republicans. But if you were membership chairperson and the membership grew by a measurable amount, for example, then you may want to consider including it. But include this information only if the activity yielded a specific or quantifiable achievement.

Likewise certain personal information has no intrinsic value, either, in terms of helping you get to the interview phase. No one needs to know your social security number or your driver's license number, for example. There is no need to risk identity theft by being overly forthcoming with this information. After all, you have no idea where this résumé will be stored and who will see it. Likewise, hobbies have no place in a résumé. If it comes up during the interview, fine, but no one needs to know you own the all-time scoring record for Words With Friends or that you like to fly kites on weekends.

Finally, physical characteristics do not belong in a résumé. People considering you for a job do not need to know your height or weight, or that one leg is longer than the other, or anything else that describes you physically. It is not relevant.

Bad Grammar, Esoteric Words, and Goofy Contact Information

Obviously, this document should command the highest level of detail you can muster. Have a friend—have several friends—review it to be sure you have not included something like "Analytic thinker and problem solvent." You should also avoid phrases such as "elucidated analysis to senior managers," when "presented" would be the better choice. I cannot over-emphasize that you should be certain you understand the meaning of the words you use, such as "Improvised the Access database" when you actually "improved" it. Finally, if you have an e-mail address like partygirl@notsobright.com or budsbestfriend@drunk.com, do not use it in your résumé. It is important to include a special note here using the proper tense of verbs. In "Work Experience," when an entry is something that is not ongoing and that was completed previously, use the past tense. If the entry describes what you are currently doing on the job (or in the internship) then use the present tense.

Objective

This is a pointless addition to a résumé for one of two reasons. In order for you to be included in the broadest possible parameters for a job—in other words to improve your odds—the objective will need to be written in such broad terms that it will literally have no meaning and will just take up valuable space on your résumé. Conversely, using your handy laptop, if you amend it to suit each job for which you apply, what does it say? It says to the reviewer that you know how to cut and paste. It also says what you should have said in your cover letter. Objectives are limiting. If you write an objective that says something like "To be in a position where I can use my analytical and interpersonal skills" and the job is for an entry level analyst, the reviewer may well conclude you are not the right person for the job because his emphasis is on analysis. Since you want to both analyze and be with people, he may conclude you would not be happy because this job is more analytic than people oriented. What he may not know is that you included *interpersonal* because you know health care organizations are always looking for people who can work in teams and you thought that *interpersonal* would reflect that notion. In short, an objective of any kind simply is not helpful; all it really does is slow the reviewer down. If you feel like you must have one, keep it bland. Above all else, avoid outlandish objectives like, "To be president of the United States."

References

There is no need to include references with your application unless specifically instructed to do so by the prospective employer. "Huh?" you say? That is correct. Do not include references with your résumé. If you say anything at all about this, there should be a line at the very bottom of the résumé (not the bottom of the page, but the last entry on the résumé) that says "References Available on Request." There is no reason to expose your references to each and every job application you make. You will be wasting the resource. Typically (but not always), the current practice is that prospective employers only call references as the last step before they offer the job. At that point, they are merely looking for validators of what they have observed, so there is no reason to litter the reviewers' desks with more than they need early in the process. If they want to call references earlier in the process, they will ask you for their information.

Before you even think about supplying references, indeed, before you even mail out a résumé, you should know what names you want to put on that list. Beyond that, however, you need to talk to the people associated with that name. You need to ask their permission to list them as a reference. Be clear about this. Do not—ever—include someone as a reference without their prior approval.

References should be listed on a separate page. Again, use the same font and stationery as the résumé and cover letter. Make the list as *clean* looking as you can; perhaps include a heading in bold such as **References for Donald L. DuRight.** As a matter of style, perhaps centering everything on the page would look good. You may want to consider doing the same kinds of things you have done on the cover letter and résumé. Here, that would mean putting the individual's name in bold and their title in italics. In addition, in a slightly smaller font that you use for the actual entry, tell—briefly—how the reference knows you. Unless there is a specific request for a personal reference, keep the references professional. No one wants to talk to your fraternity brother or your colleague from the Spanish Club.

Remember that your references are people. Do not ask someone to serve as a reference for you unless you are confident of the fact that you have a positive relationship with them and that they will support your efforts. A simple "Mr. Jones, I am starting my job search and I was wondering if it would be possible for you to serve as a positive reference for me?" will accomplish this. Note the inclusion of the word *positive*. If the person to whom you have addressed this question seems hesitant in response, then read between the lines, the answer is "no" regardless of what comes from his mouth.

Maintain a positive relationship with your references. Do not waste their time by calling and sharing every little detail about how your Skype interview went, or that you put 30 applications in the mail that morning. They do not need to know all that. Send them an e-mail from time to time to let them know how your job search is progressing. If and when you get to that critical stage with the employer saying, "The last thing we need before making you a formal offer is to talk with some of your references," (a) have the list ready and (b) give your references fair warning that they are about to receive a call from your prospective employer.

Faux Achievements

No one will be swayed by the fact that you were Miss Bigtimeuniversity or your fraternity's arm-wrestling champion. These are not accomplishments. Or if you were merely a member of anything—this is not an achievement. If you must include some of this type of material, have an "Activities" section, but keep it brief. In "Achievements," limit the entries to community, professional, and service organization awards. This business of faux achievements is a serious issue, discussed in detail in the next section.

False Information

There is no excuse—none—for including false information on your résumé. Some might see this as merely embellishing; others might see it as something *everyone* does. Both ideas could not be more incorrect. This is an issue of character and of truth telling. Here are a few examples:

1. *Radio Shack CEO Dave Edmondson* claimed to have degrees in both Psychology and Theology from Pacific Baptist College. When the *Fort Worth Star-Telegram* broke the story that he never graduated from the college, he resigned his position.
2. *Yahoo Chief Executive Scott Thompson* was found, by a New York hedge fund manager, Daniel Loeb, not to have the computer science degree he claimed to have. He had been named CEO in January 2012; Yahoo confirmed the misrepresentation on May 3, 2012. He resigned on May 13, 2012.
3. *FEMA Director Michael Brown* was closely scrutinized in the wake of his agency's mishandling of the response to Hurricane Katrina. It seems he had never been in charge of emergency services in Edmund, Oklahoma nor had he ever been a political science professor at the University of Central Oklahoma, both of which were entries on his résumé.
4. *Notre Dame Football Coach George O'Leary* had indicated he received his master's degree in education from NYU and that he had played at the University of New Hampshire. He had indeed attended NYU, but never finished the degree. And not only had he not lettered at UNH, but he never even played in a game. His tenure at Notre Dame was only five days.
5. *MIT Director of Admissions Marilee Jones* allegedly claimed to have had both a bachelor's and master's degree while working at MIT for 28 years. She left her position after it was learned that she held neither degree (Safani, 2011).

These are but five examples of people who have lied about their credentials. There are many others. But, as you can see, there are seriously negative consequences when the perfidy is discovered. In most cases, it is indeed uncovered. Yes, all of these people have gone on to other phases in their professional lives, but not before experiencing a very public humiliation when their true character was revealed. They had a few things that you do not possess, so bouncing back might have been a bit more possible for them than it would be for you at this juncture. They all had either money, experience, celebrity, or expertise, so yes, some were able to weather the storm and survive. You on the other hand are just starting on your career path; if you get caught in a material falsehood regarding your academic or employment history, the consequence would likely, relatively speaking, be much more severe.

EXAMPLES AND SOME ADDITIONAL GUIDELINES

As you look at the examples that follow, keep in mind there is, like the header for your cover letter, no one right way to construct a résumé. There are some basic guidelines:

1. Use formatting that invites the reader to take a look and makes it easy to read and find the important pieces of information.
2. Use action verbs to describe what you have done or are doing.

3. Use bullets, not paragraphs. The reader is looking for your *accomplishments*, not a job description.

4. Include and be consistent in how you treat geographic locations and dates.

5. Quantify wherever possible. Be specific in describing your achievements.

6. Spell everything correctly and use good grammar.

7. Include, and be accurate about, dates.

8. Use a chronological format—most recent first—in both the "Education" and "Employment Experience" sections.

9. Use good section headings; place "Education" first (since that is your primary accomplishment to date), followed by "Employment Experience" and then other sections as appropriate.

10. Keep it brief.

11. Make certain your contact information is correct (and remember to change your e-mail address if you use a goofy handle now).

12. Include a brief description of your prior employers (even internships).

13. Do not use the third person pronoun in your résumé.

These basic rules, combined with the material discussed above, should guide you to a complete, accurate, summary of your educational and work experiences that is easy for the reviewer to read.

The résumé shown in Figure 6-1 is a good example of what an undergraduate résumé might look like.

It has a clean format and includes geographic references and dates. Note the description of the employers—use a smaller font for this as was done here. This information is not really a highlight, but a helpful bit of information for the reader. Also notice the use of bullets to describe what she did on those various jobs. Also take note of the *active* verbs used to describe her accomplishments.

Figure 6-2 is a good example of what an MHA résumé might contain. Notice it is slightly longer and includes more material, which is natural since the person is a bit older than the undergrad and has had time to accomplish a bit more in the way of both work and education.

This person has not only been an excellent student, but an active member of the community as well. This makes a second point. This individual serves as a reminder that volunteering, especially volunteering in a way that is relevant to your academic work is not only a way to leverage your education, but also works to improve your level of experience. This résumé appears somewhat busy, but it should, given the amount of work this individual has done. Over time, she will likely want to eliminate or consolidate several of the bullet points to keep the résumé length at two pages for the first segment of her career.

To give you some additional ideas for "letterhead" or "headers" for *both* your résumé and cover letter, see Figures 6-3 and 6-4.

Figure 6-3 is a version of the name on the left with the contact information divided between the left and the right sides of the heading. This is a good look, as was mentioned in Chapter 5. Figure 6-4 is a variation on both styles, blending centering the name and separating the contact information to the left and right sides, based on academic home and permanent home.

Figures 6-5 and 6-6 all provide examples of what *not* to do. Figure 6-5, while still a very attractive looking résumé, should have common spacing among the entries. Figure 6-6 has so many mistakes one does not know where to start. If you merely glance at this, it gives a reasonably good appearance. As you read it, however, it seems top heavy with all the bold under "Education." Under "Experience," there is nothing to tell the reader what this person can do; these are all merely job titles. The titles themselves are not indented appropriately. Finally, the last heading is both in the wrong format—it should be bold—and includes a misspelled word. Also, on the second page of Figure 6-6, the writer omitted his name from the second page. This is critically important. Because résumés are never stapled, the possibility of page separation is significant. If someone opens a window and the resulting wind scatters the pages all over the floor, then the reviewer can easily reassemble the résumés that have a second page that includes the name of the applicant.

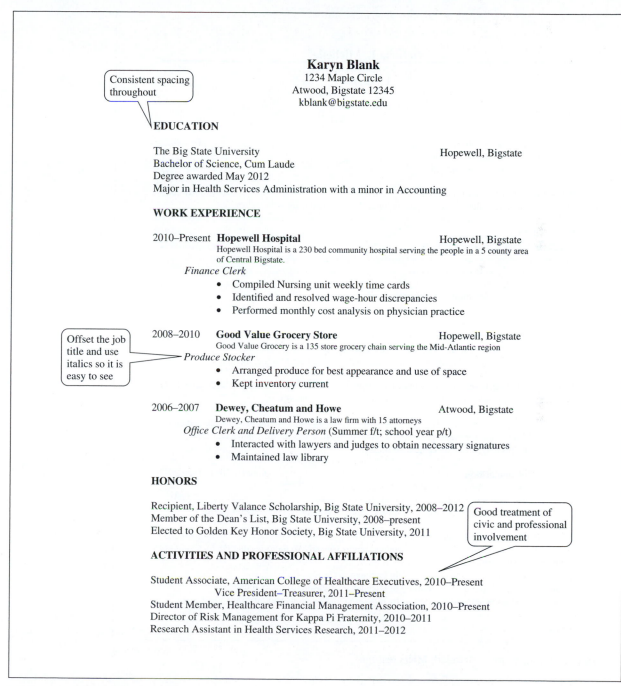

Karyn Blank
1234 Maple Circle
Atwood, Bigstate 12345
kblank@bigstate.edu

Consistent spacing throughout

EDUCATION

The Big State University   Hopewell, Bigstate
Bachelor of Science, Cum Laude
Degree awarded May 2012
Major in Health Services Administration with a minor in Accounting

WORK EXPERIENCE

2010–Present **Hopewell Hospital**   Hopewell, Bigstate
               Hopewell Hospital is a 230 bed community hospital serving the people in a 5 county area
               of Central Bigstate.
       Finance Clerk
               • Compiled Nursing unit weekly time cards
               • Identified and resolved wage-hour discrepancies
               • Performed monthly cost analysis on physician practice

2008–2010   **Good Value Grocery Store**   Hopewell, Bigstate
               Good Value Grocery is a 135 store grocery chain serving the Mid-Atlantic region
       Produce Stocker
               • Arranged produce for best appearance and use of space
               • Kept inventory current

Offset the job title and use italics so it is easy to see

2006–2007   **Dewey, Cheatum and Howe**   Atwood, Bigstate
               Dewey, Cheatum and Howe is a law firm with 15 attorneys
       Office Clerk and Delivery Person (Summer f/t; school year p/t)
               • Interacted with lawyers and judges to obtain necessary signatures
               • Maintained law library

HONORS

Recipient, Liberty Valance Scholarship, Big State University, 2008–2012
Member of the Dean's List, Big State University, 2008–present
Elected to Golden Key Honor Society, Big State University, 2011

Good treatment of civic and professional involvement

ACTIVITIES AND PROFESSIONAL AFFILIATIONS

Student Associate, American College of Healthcare Executives, 2010–Present
               Vice President–Treasurer, 2011–Present
Student Member, Healthcare Financial Management Association, 2010–Present
Director of Risk Management for Kappa Pi Fraternity, 2010–2011
Research Assistant in Health Services Research, 2011–2012

Figure 6-1 An undergraduate résumé.

Victoria L. Michelle

1755 Middlesex Rd.
Unit 6115
University City, KS 69412
michell@usml.edu
Tel: 555-843-9621

EDUCATION
University of Health Sciences, University City, KS   *May, 2012*
Masters in Health Administration
GPA: 3.77/4.0, degree anticipated

Private University, Middleville, OK   *May 2010*
Individualized Curriculum Program- Bachelor of Arts in Healthcare Administration

EXPERIENCE
Cardinal James, University City, KS   *May–July 2011*
Non-profit, continuing care retirement community. Offers independent living, assisted living, memory support, and healthcare center.
Administrative Intern
- Investigated feasibility of companion care department
- Created measurement tool to track fall and infection data as well as calculate rates
- Initiated recommendation for installation of near-miss event tracking system
- Initiated a booklet to ease funeral preplanning process
- Helped transition from paper charts to electronic records
- Participated in weekly directors meetings and organizational budget meetings

University of Health Sciences Hospital, University City, KS   *January 2011–April 2011*
700-bed academic medical center, Kansas's largest medical complex.
Administrative Intern
- Researched feasibility and offered detailed recommendations to implement telemedicine system to monitor blood glucose and blood pressure levels for the transplant center
- System is currently undergoing adoption

CLARION Competition   *January 2011–April 2011*
University of Health Sciences Local Case Competition-placed 1st
National Case Competition (University of Minnesota)-placed 2nd
- Interprofessional team case competition centered around systems-based practice

Miller St. Mary's Healthcare, University City, KS   *October 2010–April 2011*
Non-profit, 657-bed healthcare system. Includes approximately 90 facilities and doctors' offices.
Administrative Intern
- Assisted the Director of Leadership Excellence
- Served in updating the "Journey to Excellence" website for internal use
- Gained knowledge and expertise by observing presentations and meetings

(continues)

Figure 6–2 A longer, more detailed, MHA résumé.

Michelle – page 2

Dialysis Service, Inc., Hometown, OK   *September 2010–April 2011*
Non-profit corporation with over 210 ambulatory care dialysis facilities in 27 states, 7 of which are located in Hometown, OK
- Examined internal operational challenges
- Determined root causes of increased high turnover rate
- Offered detailed recommendations to create a more effective and efficient organization
- Followed up and interviewed employees to examine results of implementing recommendations

Bakeland Economic Development Council, Landlocked, OK   *May 2010–July 2010*
- Introduced local new hires and interns to the city
- Organized, coordinated, and implemented weekly tours to showcase the city

Field Work in Medicine, Middleville, OK   *August 2009–December 2009*
- Cycled through 11 clinical rotations for a semester with focus on medical ethics and medical sociology

North Hometown Hospital, Middleville, OK   *May 2009–July 2009*
45-bed, long-term acute care facility. One of five campuses of the Greenville Hospital System
- Created an action plan to improve specific opportunities
- Generated capital forecast for the following fiscal year
- Created a list of cost/savings initiatives and revenue enhancements

COMMUNITY INVOLVEMENT
UHS Heart Health   *October 2010–Present*
- Organized and planned exercise activities for patients of the UHS Heart program

Junior Doctors of Health   *September 2010–November 2010*
- Led activities for a 3rd grade class, teaching healthy lifestyle choices
- Instructed students in how to create food logs and prepare healthy snacks

ACTIVITIES
Volunteer Chair, MHA Student Government Association   *April 2011–Present*
Student Associate, American College of Healthcare Executives   *January 2011–Present*
Honor Council, College of Health Professions   *September 2011–Present*

Figure 6-2 A longer, more detailed, MHA résumé.

THE HEADINGS

This discussion would not be complete without some comment regarding the headings to use in your résumé and where to place them. The questions usually center on how to list "Experiences" or where to place "Education."

The question of where to list "education" seems pretty straight forward given that you are either doing this in preparation for a job search as you finish college or an MHA program: Education should be the first thing the reviewer sees. At this stage in your life, it is your *most significant* experience, unless you are that rare person who sailed around the globe at 16 or flew an airplane solo at the age of 12. (See the earlier discussion on hobbies.) Some would suggest "Education" should appear later in the résumé because the prospective employer is looking for experiences and wants to see what you have done. While this is true, again, your completion of college or your MHA *is* the big deal you need to promote right now. Later in life, it may be appropriate for you to reverse the order, or even change the format. For now, however, "Education" should be at the top.

The question surrounding Experience can be a bit more nuanced. You will notice in Figure 6-1, she uses the reference "Work Experience." Indeed, all of her experiences were paid jobs. Note, however, in Figure 6-2 the reference is to "Experience." This is a broader category that includes both paid and unpaid experiences. Further, in this particular—very special—case, the student included a nationally prestigious competition in which she did well, which is appropriate given the broader heading and the prestige of the event. For those who have both paid and unpaid experiences, this is a good approach to conveying the information. There is, however, another option.

You may have acquired a good bit of health care experience, but still need to list other employment. In this case, perhaps, the heading "Health Care Experience" would be useful, followed by "Other Experience." If the other experiences were all work while you were helping to pay your way through school, you may want to say "Other Work Experiences." Do not use "Professional Experience" in this category unless you are a returning adult student who actually has professional experience.

Joel J. Dullsilver
Jjd232@university.edu
555-262-3842

478 E. Sharka Avenue #422
Collegeville, PA 16801

Figure 6–3 Example of letterhead for a résumé or cover letter.

Ashley D. Winner
adw123@mailbox.com

Temporary Address
309 E. Shark Avenue
Collegeville, PA 16801
(570) 457-1450

Permanent Address
518 West Mainly Street
Orwigsburg, PA 17961
(570) 987-3899

Figure 6–4 Another example of letterhead, which blends the centering of the name and separating contact information to the left and right sides.

Sianne Drannon
1234 Health Care Circle
Hospital, Pennsylvania 12345
Residence: (123)234-2345
Cell: (345)456-5678

EDUCATION

Major University, Campground, Pennsylvania
Masters of Science in Health Administration
Degree Expected May 2006

University of Hospital School of Law, Hospital, Pennsylvania
Juris Doctorate
Degree Awarded May 2002

Bigtime State University, University City, Maryland
Bachelor of Science, *Cum Laude*
December 1998
Double Major in History and Art

> This makes good use of white space and presents a good look. However, the indentations from the entries under "Education" are different from the indentations of "Work Experience." These should be the same.

WORK EXPERIENCE

2003–Present   Clarion University Health System, Office of the Chief Executive Officer
Clarion, Pennsylvania
Graduate Administrative Assistant

2003   Wellbe County Economic & Industrial Development Authority
Pelham, Alabama
Project Manager

2000–2002   Dewey, Cheatum & Howe, Attorneys-at-Law
Goodtimes, Alabama
Law Clerk

2001   Pennsylvania Attorney General, Criminal Division
Harrisburg, Pensylvania
Law Clerk

2001   U.S. Senator Albert Morse (PA)
Judiciary Subcommittee on Administrative Oversight and the Courts
Washington, D.C.
Law Clerk

2000   The Honorable William J. Bryant, Federal District Judge
Harrisburg, Pennsylvania
Legal Intern

2000   Pennsylvania Supreme Court
Harrisburg, Pennsylvania
Legal Intern

Figure 6–5 An example without common spacing throughout the entries.   *(continues)*

HONORS, ACTIVITIES AND PROFESSIONAL AFFILIATIONS

Recipient, Magnolia Regional Health Center Auxiliary Scholarship, 2003–2004.
Justice, Honor Court, University of Pittsburgh School of Law, 2001–2002.
Member, Bench & Bar Legal Honor Society, 2001–2002.
Recipient, Pittsburgh Circuit Judges' Scholarship, 2000–2001.
Recognized in The National Dean's List, 1998–1999.
Junior editor, Law & Psychology Review, 2001–2002.
Participant, Volunteer Lawyers' Program, 2000–2001.
Student Associate, American College of Healthcare Executives, 2003–present.
Student Member, Healthcare Financial Management Association, 2003–present.
Member, Pennsylvania Bar Association, 2002–present.

Figure 6–5 An example without common spacing throughout the entries.

For anyone else, this is a misleading overstatement. You should use these separate, distinct headings *only* if you have amassed a great deal of experience. The person whose résumé is Figure 6-2 comes close to benefitting from multiple "Experience" headings. Even here, however, keeping it simple works. A generic "Experience" is the best approach as a graduating student.

Beneath those headings, all of the entries should be chronological with most recent at the top and proceeding down the page the farther back in time as you move down through the list. These entries should include name of organization; brief description of the organization; the dates you were there; and the title you held. Beneath all of that, you should have bullet points that briefly describe what you did. Figures 6-1 and 6-2 both have good examples of this.

After "Education" and "Experience," the choices become a bit more specific to the person. If you have gleaned a host of honors and recognition, then an "Honors" heading might be appropriate. If you have been an active volunteer in on-campus activity, then "Student Activities" or "Cocurricular Activities" might be appropriate. If you have been active both on and off campus as a volunteer, you may want to consider something like what the author did in Figure 6-2 with "Community Involvement" and "Activities."

The purposes of an "Education" heading and an "Experience" heading are self-evident. Demonstrate academic qualifications and highlight accomplishments that make you the right choice for the job. After that, "Honors" or "Activities" are there to demonstrate some degree of life balance. Part of being professional is contributing time, talent, or treasure back to the community, whether it is the community where you live, or your community of professionals, or both. Life-balance is about doing something outside the sphere of work that you enjoy. So while things like golf or other hobbies like being a gamer are not particularly germane to your status as a professional, and thus to the résumé, demonstrating some level of interest in the community beyond yourself most certainly is important for the reviewer to know. If you are active in Habitat for Humanity or Meals on Wheels or a disease charity, your résumé should reflect that important fact.

ORDER OF THE CONTENT

The content within each of the headings should *always*, without exception, be listed chronologically with the most recent entry on top, followed by successive entries going back in time. Sometimes things may overlap and that is OK. Your most recent experience is the most relevant; hence, it should always

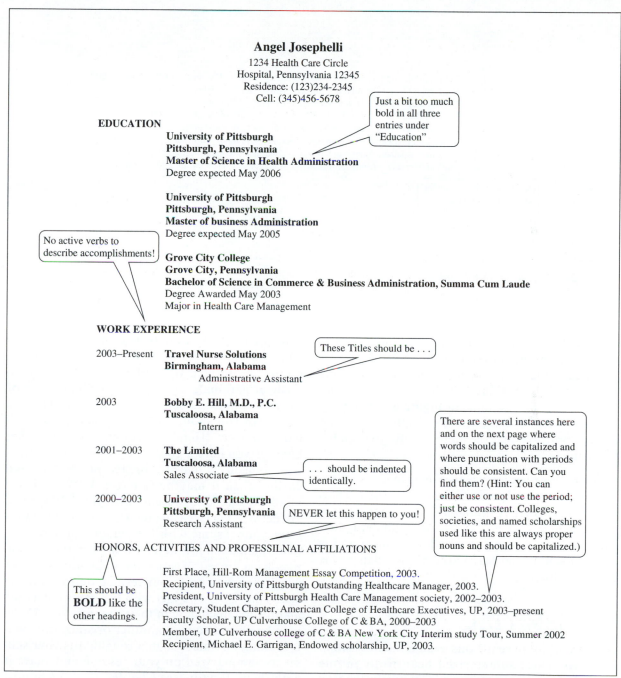

Angel Josephelli
1234 Health Care Circle
Hospital, Pennsylvania 12345
Residence: (123)234-2345
Cell: (345)456-5678

> Just a bit too much bold in all three entries under "Education"

EDUCATION

University of Pittsburgh
Pittsburgh, Pennsylvania
Master of Science in Health Administration
Degree expected May 2006

University of Pittsburgh
Pittsburgh, Pennsylvania
Master of business Administration
Degree expected May 2005

> No active verbs to describe accomplishments!

Grove City College
Grove City, Pennsylvania
Bachelor of Science in Commerce & Business Administration, Summa Cum Laude
Degree Awarded May 2003
Major in Health Care Management

WORK EXPERIENCE

2003–Present   **Travel Nurse Solutions**
               Birmingham, Alabama
               Administrative Assistant

> These Titles should be . . .

2003   **Bobby E. Hill, M.D., P.C.**
               Tuscaloosa, Alabama
               Intern

2001–2003   **The Limited**
               Tuscaloosa, Alabama
               Sales Associate

> . . . should be indented identically.

2000–2003   **University of Pittsburgh**
               Pittsburgh, Pennsylvania
               Research Assistant

> NEVER let this happen to you!

> There are several instances here and on the next page where words should be capitalized and where punctuation with periods should be consistent. Can you find them? (Hint: You can either use or not use the period; just be consistent. Colleges, societies, and named scholarships used like this are always proper nouns and should be capitalized.)

HONORS, ACTIVITIES AND PROFESSILNAL AFFILIATIONS

> This should be **BOLD** like the other headings.

First Place, Hill-Rom Management Essay Competition, 2003.
Recipient, University of Pittsburgh Outstanding Healthcare Manager, 2003.
President, University of Pittsburgh Health Care Management society, 2002–2003.
Secretary, Student Chapter, American College of Healthcare Executives, UP, 2003–present
Faculty Scholar, UP Culverhouse College of C & BA, 2000–2003
Member, UP Culverhouse college of C & BA New York City Interim study Tour, Summer 2002
Recipient, Michael E. Garrigan, Endowed scholarship, UP, 2003.

(continues)

Figure 6–6 Can you spot the errors?

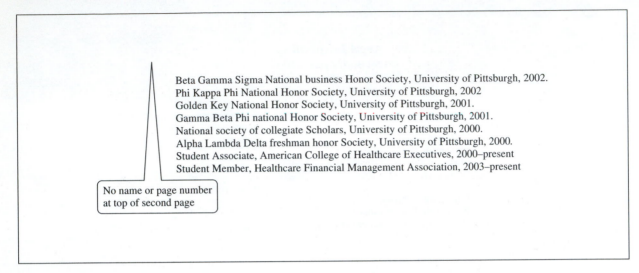

Beta Gamma Sigma National business Honor Society, University of Pittsburgh, 2002.
Phi Kappa Phi National Honor Society, University of Pittsburgh, 2002
Golden Key National Honor Society, University of Pittsburgh, 2001.
Gamma Beta Phi national Honor Society, University of Pittsburgh, 2001.
National society of collegiate Scholars, University of Pittsburgh, 2000.
Alpha Lambda Delta freshman honor Society, University of Pittsburgh, 2000.
Student Associate, American College of Healthcare Executives, 2000–present
Student Member, Healthcare Financial Management Association, 2003–present

No name or page number at top of second page

Figure 6–6 Can you spot the errors?

be first. As you can see in Figures 6-1 and 6-2, specific treatment of dates can be done several ways. In either case, the reviewer can capture the important information by reading left to right on only one or two lines. The example in Figure 6-2 is slightly better because it includes months, following the general principle that the more specific you can be, the better.

Finally, the question whether to include your GPA in the "Education" section is one that is pretty common. The answer is simple: If your grades are an asset, include it; if not, don't. As a standard, anything above 3.5 on a 4.0 scale for an undergrad is a clear asset; for an MHA student, the standard is probably closer to 3.75.

TRANSMITTAL

Now that you have all this accumulated wisdom and experience summarized beautifully in one place, how do you circulate it? Obviously, the first answer is with your cover letter when applying for a known job or position. Second, you always carry three or four copies with you. You never know who you might encounter who is willing, and in a position, to help your job search. Third, obviously at national, regional, or local meetings of the professional association you joined. This does not mean you should walk up, shake someone's hand, and say "Here's my résumé." On the other hand, if you have a good fairly long conversation with someone at one of those receptions discussed earlier, then it may be fair to ask "Would you mind if I shared my résumé with you?" When you are networking (see Chapter 4), you should always leave your résumé with the person you have visited. Again, you just never know when that person may have a need of someone with your skills or when they may pass your résumé on to someone else. That COO you met with last month may see an opening upcoming in their organization. Or he may know someone in another organization who is looking for someone that roughly fits your skill set as summarized on your résumé and share it with them. Finally (see Chapter 2), you can post the bulk of your résumé on LinkedIn, which will increase the exposure it receives exponentially.

TABLE OF ACTION VERBS

TABLE 6–1: **A Partial List of Action Verbs**

Acted	Communicated	Empathized	Handled	Logged
Adapted	Compared	Enforced	Headed	Made
Addressed	Completed	Established	Helped	Maintained
Administered	Computed	Estimated	Identified	Managed
Advised	Conceived	Evaluated	Illustrated	Manipulated
Allocated	Copied	Examined	Imagined	Mediated
Analyzed	Counseled	Expanded	Implemented	Memorized
Approved	Created	Experimented	Improved	Monitored
Arranged	Dealt	Extracted	Improvised	Met
Ascertained	Decided	Facilitated	Increased	Modeled
Assisted	Defined	Filed	Indexed	Observed
Attained	Delegated	Financed	Initiated	Obtained
Audited	Delivered	Fixed	Inspected	Offered
Brought	Designed	Followed	Investigated	Operated
Budgeted	Detected	Formulated	Judged	Ordered
Calculated	Directed	Gathered	Kept	Performed
Chartered	Documented	Gave	Learned	Received
Checked	Drove	Generated	Lectured	Taught
Classified	Dug	Got	Led	Utilized
Coached	Edited	Governed	Lifted	Volunteered
Collected	Eliminated	Guided	Listened	Worked

CONCLUSION

By now you should realize that there is no *one* magical way to create a résumé, but rather the creation of a résumé should be a snapshot of your life, presented in an easy-to-read format that casts your work in a favorable light without falsifying any information. While there is no one special format, there are several rules and guidelines about the overall look and specific content of the résumé. Like everything else in this book, the résumé is about you, and therefore, should be an accurate reflection of who you are and, more importantly, what kind of work you can do. So, the résumé needs to reflect your complete work and educational histories (starting with college) and it must be free of errors in spelling, grammar, or formatting.

Now is the time to start creating, or recreating, yours. Go to it!

Observations from the Professionals

What I Look for in a Résumé

Kyle W. Dorsey, MHA is currently the Health Center Administrator of Advanced Heart and Lung Failure at Duke University Medical Center. Duke's mission is to provide exceptional and innovative care to patients, families, and the community through the finest integration of clinical care, education, and research, while respecting the needs of the human spirit. Kyle is a graduate of The Ohio State University's MHA program.

Your résumé is the front door to your future. It is up to you how you would like to mold and paint your front door and present yourself to your potential employer. While you want your résumé to stand out from others, keep in mind it is also generally the first impression a hiring manager will have of you. It is an important opportunity for you to market your skills and accomplishments in a way that aligns with the job in a professional, yet creative way that will catch the employer's attention. On average, only 30 seconds is spent reviewing each résumé. Over the next few paragraphs, I will share attributes that lead me to spend more time considering a candidate for hire.

When reviewing résumés for a vacant position, I look for a candidate who is able to meet very basic requirements that any motivated individual would be able to meet. The résumé should be well organized and easy to read so the reviewer can quickly identify the applicant's education, professional skills, work history, community service activities, professional affiliations, honors, etc. Résumés with fonts that are difficult to read and are inconsistently structured quickly find their way to the recycle bin. Although it may sound obvious, take the time to check spelling and punctuation. I am amazed by how many résumés I have reviewed from college prepared individuals that have spelling and grammatical errors.

I review educational history first to ensure the candidate meets the minimum requirements for the vacancy (bachelor's, master's, or higher degree). I then review the individual's work history to get an idea for their historical experience and what they were able to contribute to the department/organization while in their previous roles. As you construct your résumé, under each experience, take time to structure the bullets for each position to give the reader a high-level review of your responsibilities, accomplishments, and what you were able to gain from the position.

Be cautious not to provide extraneous and/or granular detail that will overwhelm the reader. If you have minimal work experience, you will not have a several page résumé (and that is acceptable). As an example, if your only previous experience is a residency/internship, your résumé will most likely be only a page long. It is much better to keep your résumé concise rather than try to fill all the white space with "junk." Often times, the reader uses your résumé to determine how adept you are at writing and organizing thoughts. It is best to use action verbs, such as those provided in this chapter, accurately to clearly articulate your accomplishments and highlight the reasons you would be the best candidate for the new position.

In addition to reviewing the bullets under each position, I pay careful attention to the length of time the individual spent in each role. When hiring someone to join my team, it is my goal to ensure they will stay for the long run. Research has shown that teamwork and morale are higher when turnover is low and trust is high amongst members of the team. It is also very costly to continuously recruit and train new hires. That being said, I avoid interviewing applicants who hop from job to job on a regular basis without justification. It is my perception that these individuals are not loyal and will not be motivated to stay in a position when another opportunity presents itself.

Outside of your work experience, I am also very interested in your skills and extracurricular accomplishments. This part of your résumé is your opportunity to standout from others. If you are involved with any professional networks, list them so the reader knows you are taking personal time to advance your career and get involved with the community. In addition to benefiting you, it will benefit the organization if they have employees represented on community boards and are giving backing to social organizations. In addition, if you received any academic or professional awards or certifications, share them with the reader. This is not the time to share that you were the "Flip Cup Champion" of your fraternity. While this example may be rash, be careful not to list any political, religious, or social affiliations that may be controversial with the interviewer. Only share examples that help you further demonstrate why you are the best candidate.

When actively seeking a new position, it is appropriate to have different résumés for different opportunities. You will want to tailor your résumé to be more specific for each position you are interested in, and this is perfectly acceptable. Truthfully update your experiences so they directly correlate with the needs and requirements of the new job opening.

To help ensure your résumé is clearly organized and structured appropriately, ask several trustworthy individuals to review and provide candid feedback. If you know someone close to the position for which you are applying, it would be advantageous to also ask him or her to provide feedback on your résumé. Do not feel obligated to accept every edit that is shared with you. It is more important for you to feel comfortable with your résumé and the words you have chosen to represent yourself. However, it is a positive experience to hear what others think and their perception of the words you chose to represent you.

As you work on your résumé, put yourself in the hiring manager's position and think about what characteristics you would be looking for in the position. Then, focus your attention on creatively and succinctly meeting this need. By being organized and choosing appropriate action verbs to describe your accomplishments to date, you will be taking the steps needed to move your résumé to the top of the stack and will soon be receiving a contact to setup an interview.

EXERCISES

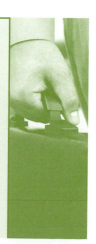

6-1. This is a good time to re-visit the question of which font to use. Look at your cover letter and the letterhead. Do you think the letterhead reflects the look you want? Exchange your letterhead with a partner. Review and critique for "clean" look and style. If you adopt a different "résumé" head here, be sure to also change the letterhead for your cover letter. But if you are satisfied with the letterhead you have already created, and want to use it as your "résumé" head, start constructing your résumé by putting it at the top of the page.

6-2. Insert headings for "Education" and "Experiences" and another category you decide from the discussion earlier in the chapter.

6-3. List the name of your college, the city in which it is located and your degree. If you have not yet graduated, insert "degree anticipated" as seen in Figure 6-2. If you are in an MHA program, repeat the process with the graduate degree on top. Next, make a list of all the jobs, internships, and significant (extending over a period of time) volunteer experiences you have had. Put them in chronological order and list the dates beside each. Edit and make certain the information is accurate.

6-4. Transfer the information from Exercise 6-3 into the template you created in Exercise 6-2. Complete the information for the third category. Get a partner; exchange résumés; and, provide each other detailed, critical feedback about the résumé.

BIBLIOGRAPHY

Safani, B. (2011, January 26). *AOL Jobs Week*. Retrieved May 15, 2012, from Lying to Get a Job: Nine Famous Fibbers: http://www.job.aol.com

Chapter 7

Getting to the "On-Site" Interview: Application Is in the Mail, Now What?

Now that your perfect cover letter and terrific résumé are in the mail you just sit back and wait for the offers to roll in, right? Not so much. Let us call this the pre-interview stage. For much of this part of the process, you have no control. That is why it was so important to have the cover letter and the résumé just exactly right, because now, for the most part, events over which you have no control will take place. There are some things you can do, however, during this period that might help your chances of getting to the on-site interview.

At the end of this chapter, students will understand how to relate well to those who are coordinating the search; will understand how to handle a phone interview and a Skype interview; will appreciate the importance of doing additional research on the prospective employer; and will understand how to follow up on the application that has not yet been given an acknowledgement.

NO NAIL BITING, PLEASE

At this juncture you have pretty much done everything you can do to get an interview. You have an excellent cover letter and outstanding résumé. There is no need, however, to worry about whether you will or will not get an on-site, or even a telephone, interview. This is true for one simple reason: It will not

do any good. This is simply out of your hands, so all the worry and stress in the world will not help. If you paid attention the last four or six years in school, got decent grades, did a noteworthy amount of legitimate volunteer professional-related experiences, and packaged it all nicely in your application, then you have done everything you can and, as the old saw goes: "It is what it is." On the other hand, if you have been a slacker riding on the coattails of your classmates, majored in social events instead of health administration, and do not have much on your résumé, it will not do you any good to worry, either. Your chances are negligible; again, "It is what it is."

THE NEXT STEPS

Whether you are an undergrad applying for a posted job opening or an MHA student applying for a residency or fellowship (or a posted job vacancy), you have a right to know if your application was received. The good employers will send some kind of acknowledgment. This will be a neutral document or an e-mail that merely states the organization has received your application. Sometimes, however, whoever is coordinating the process may get caught up in other details and will not send such an acknowledgment. This may be the organization's practice; it may be that the person simply was overwhelmed with work and did not find the time to let you know your application had arrived. You will not know the reason, and frankly, it does not matter. There is, however, something you can do about this state of affairs.

If you mail your application on a Monday, you can generally assume it was received on Wednesday or Thursday at the latest. If you submitted electronically, then it was received contemporaneously with your upload. The days are important, because if you have not received an acknowledgement within 10 days or so *from the date of receipt*, a follow up telephone call is appropriate.

This will be an important call. You will be speaking with the boss's assistant, the current fellow or resident, or an HR representative. You should assume that the substance of your conversation will be shared with those making the decision regarding the position. (It may or may not be, but you should assume that it is; turn this into another opportunity to market your skills.)

Call the contact person listed in the ad or other materials about the position. Again, put on your very best manners: At this point, you are selling, not buying, so demonstrate a high level of emotional intelligence and restrain from exhibiting whatever stress or frustration you may feel. The question to the contact person goes something like this:

"Ms. Smith, this is Donald DuRight. How are you?"

She gives a polite response indicating she's fine, rather than bore you with the fact that she got no sleep because the baby was fussy all night and how her car broke down that morning making her late for work and now she's behind on *everything*, but seems just a tad bit abrupt when she says, "I'm fine, Donald, how can I help you?"

"I'm calling to make sure you received my application. I sent it about two weeks ago and just wanted to make certain you received it and were aware of my interest in the position." Note—there is no reference to the prospective employer's poor behavior of not sending an acknowledgment; simply not politic in this context. And perhaps something for you to keep in mind as you explore whether that is the place you want to work.

"Yes, Donald, we did receive it and the committee is reviewing it along with all the applications to narrow down the pool."

"Good, thank you. I'm glad to know I'm still being considered. Would you happen to have any insight you could share regarding the timetable?"

"All I know, Donald, is that the committee is meeting later this week and will select a number of people for Skype interviews."

"That's good to know, Ms. Smith. I appreciate your sharing that with me. Thank you for your time and have a great day."

"You're welcome, Donald. Good luck and thanks for calling."

So, you just had a chance to remind a key person in the process that you are interested *and* you learned a little bit about the organization's selection process and timetable. Why is this important? Well, if you have—and you should have—other applications pending, you may need to coordinate the timing of interviews. If you are really lucky, you will have the opportunity to coordinate more than one interview; and if you are *really* lucky perhaps more than one offer.

This is about as much as you can control at this point. There may be a need for an additional follow up call for some reason, but that would be rare. You do not want to appear to be begging, or desperate, nor do you want to make a nuisance of yourself.

There is one exception to this process and that is the electronic application. It seems that the electronic application process is depersonalizing in several ways, one of which includes not acknowledging the application's receipt. This means it is up to you whether you want to pursue affirmation of the application's receipt.

NEXT STEP: THE TELEPHONE INTERVIEW

Monday morning of the next week, Ms. Smith calls you on your cell phone while you are in class. Fortunately, you have already changed the voice mail greeting from "Yo, dude, w'ssup. Can't gab now, but will hit ya' back later" to the admittedly less fun and more sedate: "You have reached the voice mail for Donald DuRight. I am not able to take your call at the moment, but please leave your name and number; I will call as soon as I am able." It should go without saying—but I will say it anyway—change the goofy greeting on your voice mail to something that sounds like the young professional you are in the process of becoming.

When you return her call later on Monday morning, Ms. Smith informs you that you have been selected for a telephone interview. Because there were so many applicants, the committee decided to interview a number of candidates by phone and then several of those will be selected for a Skype interview. Of course, you express to her how pleased you are to be selected for this next step in the process and proceed to schedule a phone interview for the coming Thursday morning. (Note: For undergrads, this interview is likely to be with the hiring manager and perhaps a representative from human resources; or it might be just one or the other. For MHAs applying for a residency or fellowship, this will most likely be the current resident or fellow and another person.)

Note the time and day for the interview. Be certain you understand the time of day for the interview, particularly if the prospective employer is in a different time zone. Almost nothing could be worse than agreeing on "3 PM," when you are thinking central time and the employer is in the eastern time zone. They called and called and called again at 3 PM while you were out jogging to calm your nerves at 2 PM in advance of your 3 PM interview. Oops. Do not blow the opportunity because you misunderstood the time zones.

At any rate, it is now Monday morning; you just scheduled the phone interview for Thursday morning. That leaves you Monday afternoon and evening, all day Tuesday and Wednesday before the big event. Is this a good time to relieve the stress by starting the weekend early and party till Wednesday night? Or maybe you think you will disconnect from classes because you have "got the job" and finish that excellent novel you have been reading. Hardly.

Interviews by telephone are somewhat awkward and, therefore, demand a lot more of the people on both ends of the line. From your perspective, you may raise your voice (not to a shout) to make a point and you will not be able to see the facial responses to confirm for you that either you had the most brilliant insight of the year, or said the dumbest thing these people have ever heard. There is no visual feedback for either extreme; no validation to assure you that you are on the right path. Partly for this reason, you will need to double down on your preparation and how you express yourself.

This is the time to prepare. Think about an interview and what they will want to know about you. How do you organize this preparation? What does the employer want to accomplish during this session?

Given that our scenario is a telephone interview with 12 candidates to pare the number down to three for a Skype interview, this is a preliminary screening interview. The employer is looking for disqualifiers. That is to say, the employer is looking for reasons the candidate will not be a good fit with the organization. This could be anything from GPA to a preference for a particular strength or interest of the candidate.

The questions you will most likely face are below. But to be clear, this is not an *exclusive* list of questions. There could be, and you should assume there will be, others. This list, however, represents the questions you will be most likely to hear:

1. Tell us about yourself.
2. What do you know about our organization?
3. Why do you want to be a <insert health care sector of interest to you>?
4. Where do you see yourself in three to five years?

Those four questions could very well tell the employer enough about you and the other candidates that they will be able to winnow down the candidates from 12 to 3. This should guide your preparation.

Tell Us about Yourself

This is where you will use your elevator speech or something you have developed from your elevator speech. Review Chapter 4 and Chapter 1 if you need to; however, here is where you want to provide a brief, verbal picture of yourself. Do not read from your résumé; the caller is looking at it and can read perfectly well. Amplify on the content in the résumé. Give them an idea of who you are and what you are capable of doing. Use your voice to paint a picture of you; let your voice show a bit of excitement over something of which you are particularly proud. If you did a great job on an interesting project over the summer, get that into the conversation. Again, no one can do this but you, so spend some time developing some points that describe you and your capabilities. Make your response as conversational as possible, meaning that you should not at this moment regurgitate a canned speech you memorized. Rather, talk conversationally about who you are and the passions you have about health care. The key to this question is that the employer is looking for your depth of commitment to the profession; how big a part does it play in your life? For undergraduates, if the health care administration major is just the path of least resistance to graduation for you, then chances are that will show in your response to this question. If you are passionate about <*insert the sector of health care industry of interest to you*> then the odds of your moving to the next step are improved.

What Do You Know about Our Organization?

Back in Chapter 3, you were asked to do some basic research about a host of organizations you were considering as possible employers. Now is the time to do a bit more research in depth. Return to the website; look for awards the organization has won or distinctions it has achieved. Make notes and commit that kind of information to memory. You might also go to Glassdoor.com and look for what current and former employees have said about the company. This is *always* instructive, as there are also ratings for CEOs, salary information, and a host of other "tidbits" about many companies. Your local hospital, of course, may not be here, but if you are considering large health care systems, or some other sector of the industry dominated by larger players (such as pharmacy or technology supplier) they may well be included here.

For your purposes, however, you want to know not only about awards, but other developments impacting on, or a product of, the organization where you are interviewing. If this is a hospital and they are building a new bed tower, be sure you know about it and comment on it during your response to this question. If it is a pharmaceutical company and they are awaiting FDA approval of a new drug, mention it or ask about it. Go beyond looking at the organization's website; Google it and see what the search uncovers. Read up-to-date news accounts of this organization and make sure you mention these developments during your response to this question. Check out *Modern Healthcare,* as well as other industry sector-related and trade publications and *U.S. News & World Report* to find awards or citations or interesting developments in their organizations. Check the local newspaper as well, as smaller more local organizations may not draw the attention of the national press.

Showing that you know something of the organization is *the most effective* way of communicating to them that you are genuinely interested in the position. And your interest level is one of the things being assessed during this interview, and in this question particularly.

Why Do You Want to Be a <Fill in the Blank>?

This again gets back to Chapter 1. Here is your opportunity to amplify on the elevator speech. While that conversation is a general overview about you and some of the things you have done, this question invites a much more focused response about your passion. For each of us, this is somewhat personal. Many people get into health care because someone in their family is some kind of health care professional or perhaps because someone in their family suffered a severe injury or illness that motivated the student to move in this direction.

Others may be attracted to the field because it is ever changing and filled with problems to be solved. Perhaps they were attracted to health care because it is an opportunity to help people. Give this some thought: Why did you choose this major? Or why did you seek an MHA? Review Chapter 1 if that would be helpful.

Whatever the reason, be certain that you are honest about why you have a passion for health care and let the conviction show through in your voice.

Where Do You See Yourself in Three to Five Years?

This is a very revealing question. While there is no right answer as, again, you need to develop your own life/career plan, there are some principles you can avoid or include, as the case may be. The question is designed to elicit your commitment to the profession and the work that goes with it. If you have an answer that focuses on being in a "good job" with "job security" and "good benefits," that may suggest to the employer that you do not want to be challenged to grow and improve. If you say, "I expect to be a vice president of an integrated health services delivery system," the employer may see that as an absence of realism and self-awareness on your part. It is, after all, a bit outlandish. The balance here is not to suggest that you expect to be in a particular position, but rather that you are in a position to make a positive contribution to your employer, one that challenges your skills and one that gives you an opportunity to grow professionally and grow within the organization.

In short, the employer is looking for someone who wants to assume increasing levels of responsibilities and make positive contributions to the organization; someone who wants to learn and grow; and someone who is ambitious, but not blindingly so.

One final thought about the telephone interview: be conversational and engaging. When answering the questions, do not ramble on and on, but respond thoroughly; be succinct and focused. If you are one who gets nervous about these kinds of conversations, get out for a run or a walk; get some exercise. Focus not on yourself, but on the organization. Think about what it would be like to be there. Paint a mental picture of yourself working there. Remember that the people asking the questions were all, at some point in one way or another, in the same position that you now occupy. Be sure to look at this step in the process as an educational experience. If this works out and you move on to the next step, terrific. If not, it certainly is not the end of the world and you should be able to take some valuable lessons from having gone through this process.

THE NEXT STEP: THE SKYPE INTERVIEW

An increasing number of employers are using Skype as an initial interview. Usually they interview several using this Internet technology. It has some advantages over the telephone interview because you can actually see the person on the other end of the phone line. The verbal exchanges may be the same—same questions, same answers. The video dimension of Skype, however, changes the dynamic in ways that call for you to pay special attention.

If you set up the monitor so you can see a small picture of yourself, and if you look at it a lot, which is an understandable temptation, you will not be looking at the interviewers. They will be seeing basically a partial profile of either the left or right side of your face, depending on how your monitor is set up. So, no matter how good looking your ears may be, either arrange the monitor so your picture does not appear, or have—and use—sufficient will power to ignore it. The obviously easy solution is to change the appearance of the monitor so you do not see yourself at all.

Second, if you look at the screen so you can see your interviewers, you again will not be looking at them—from their point of view. They will see an image of you with your eyes aimed below theirs. Only

POTENTIAL PHONE / SKYPE INTERVIEW QUESTIONS

Sample Questions

1. Tell me about yourself.
2. What do you know about our organization?
3. Why do you want to be a hospital administrator? Or why do you want to be an administrative fellow at X?
4. Where do you see yourself in three to five years?
5. How would you describe diversity and why it is important in workgroups?
6. What would your classmates say about you?
7. What is your biggest strength and weakness? Or what is your biggest weakness and how do you address it?
8. Give me an example of a time you had to overcome a challenge? Or how would you approach a colleague if they were not pulling their weight on a project?
9. If you only had enough money to purchase a brand new 64 slice CT scanner or expand your internal medicine department with three new physicians, which would you choose and why?
10. Do you really want to live in <fill in the blank—city>? (This is where I would show I did my homework about the city and was actually interested in the fellowship.)
11. What is your favorite class in your (undergrad health administration) (MHA) curriculum and why?
12. Who do you look up to?
13. What health care-related periodicals or websites do you frequently read?
14. How would you address a physician who has recently been yelling at nurses?
15. Finally, do you have any questions for us?

when you look directly into the camera will you be looking into the eyes of your interviewers, as they will be looking at the screen to see you. So, the "easier said than done" solution is to (a) look at the screen when they are asking a question, so you can at least get a visual "feel" for the meaning of the question and (b) focus your eyes exclusively on the camera in your computer when answering a question. If you do this, you will appear forthright and candid as you would be if you are interviewed in person and looked the inquisitor in the eye when you answered. The disadvantage, of course, is that you cannot directly see their faces to garner a visual "feel" for how they are receiving the answer. The best you will be able to do is to see them peripherally and hopefully that will give you a sufficient cue regarding your response.

There is, of course, an additional aspect to the video nature of Skype. In a telephone interview, you can wear last semester's jeans and a T-shirt you pulled out of the dirty laundry because you were out of clothes. Clearly, you cannot do that with Skype. Dress as if you were going to an on-site interview.

It does not matter that you will be in your bedroom at home; dress up. While you are dressing up, clean up your room or the background where you will be doing the interview. The background may well be visible, so make certain it is tidy. I have done several Skype interviews and could not help but notice some unfortunate characteristics of the room where the interviewee was sitting.

One other thought for both the telephone and Skype interviews: Find a quiet place to have this conversation. Find a place you know will be quiet for the entire hour scheduled for your interview. The last thing you need is background noise of any kind.

QUESTIONS YOU WILL LIKELY ENCOUNTER

There will be more on interview questions and answers in Chapter 8, which deals with the subject in depth. This chapter has provided the four most likely questions you will encounter in the preliminary interview, whether the interview is over the telephone or by Skype. A list of possible questions you might encounter over the phone or by Skype (or, even in an on-site interview) appears on the previous page. Note that some of these questions are about the person and some are "behavioral"—about how the person responded to certain situations. Again, this is not an exhaustive list, but rather a sample of some of the questions you most likely will be asked.

BE SURE TO SAY *THANK YOU*

This does not mean the "Thank you for your time" you say verbally at the end of your interview conversation. The handwritten thank you note on a *thank you* card or note paper is the best. Send one to everyone who participated in the interview. *Everyone*. It only takes a few minutes and it makes a remarkable and positive impression.

Some would say the e-mail thank you note is OK. It is better than nothing at all. Indeed, as we move forward in time more and more are finding e-mail sufficient and have fewer expectations of receiving a handwritten note. The increasing rarity of the handwritten note suggests that sending a written "thank you" will be noticed (in a good way) more prominently.

CONCLUSION

As you can see there are a lot of nuances to the interview process. It is about much more than being *Joe Friendly* with a knack for being able to get along with everyone from the laundry workers to the CEO (though that certainly is a great gift!). Research about the organization is the foundation to getting an interview and it is the foundation to having a successful interview. Demonstrating your own passion for being a part of the health care field, coupled with your ability to articulate current knowledge of the organization with which you are interviewing will help you stand apart from other applicants in telephone, Skype and live on-site interviews.

In brief summary: Do the homework; let your voice demonstrate a bit of variable tone to let your genuine passion for the field be known, and; for Skype interviews be sure to look at the camera, not the monitor. And most importantly, always say "Thank you" personally to everyone involved.

Observations from the Professionals

Emory Health Care Management Development Program: What We Do and What We Look for in a Candidate

Donald Brunn, MHSA, FACHE, is the president and chief operating officer of The Emory Clinic, the 1274 physician faculty practice of the Emory University School of Medicine and President of Emory Specialty Associates, the 170 physician community practice of Emory Healthcare. These physician groups serve patients in over 100 clinic locations and 7 hospitals in central and northern Georgia and represent the portal of access for Emory's health care system.

Imagine a place that invests in the next generation of health care administrators. Imagine a program established to provide new health care administration graduates with hands-on operational, budget, and people management experience at a leading academic medical center. Imagine the potential return on investment when an organization builds its future senior talent from hand-chosen, intentionally groomed and mentored graduates who hold "real" jobs while they matriculate through a formal leadership and management curriculum.

This was The Emory Clinic's vision when it founded its Management Development Program in 2004. The program is designed to prepare talent to assume key leadership roles in Emory's dynamic health care enterprise and academic/research enterprise—all serving a top-tier School of Medicine, in one of the nation's fastest growing regions. Since its inception, the program has enrolled 40 participants in full time, budgeted roles—deployed to clinical departments, business services departments, and financial services areas.

Candidates to the program are all masters-prepared individuals who are seeking their first operational or management role—aligning their administrative residency or fellowship requirements with meaningful experience in a dynamic ambulatory care and physician practice environment, but going above and beyond the scope of a traditional administrative residency or fellowship in important ways. The program's participants represent 18 distinct university masters degree programs, and hold Masters of Business Administration, Masters of Public Health, and Masters of Health Services Administration degrees. The diversity of graduate programs is matched by a commitment to recruit a diverse and balanced workgroup.

Recruitment Process: Step by Step:

1. The Emory Clinic's Office of Development Programs holds recruiting sessions each Fall and Spring semester on four to six college campuses, to spread information about the program, and to screen potential applicants—often from a pool selected by a participating school's program faculty.
2. In a typical year, up to 75 applicants complete a rigorous application packet that is intended to assess the candidate's ability to articulate their career interest, their ability to demonstrate written communication skills, and their ability to provide a compelling defense of their skill set with the program's competency profile.
3. About 20 individuals are invited to one of two on-site interview sessions, held in November and March each year. The interview sessions expose candidates to interview panels who are trained to look for mastery of project management, organizational communication, financial, and business acumen skills as well as leadership and values fit.

Three phases, six levels plus "merit badges":

1. Successful candidates are hired in two on-boarding cycles, in January and June, and are assigned to a leader (their direct supervisor) and a sponsor who serves in an executive-coach capacity for the participant. Being selected as a leader of an MDP participant is itself a rigorous process—the leader must demonstrate their commitment to the program's structured learning and evaluation process and must agree to place priority on the participant's career development and learning experience, while holding the participant accountable to produce management results.
2. MDP participants fill full-time budgeted positions that would otherwise be filled by this-job-is-my-career-destination managers. Most often, participants complete their entire program in their first, home department, but about 25% choose to rotate among departments as positions and roles become available.
3. The three phases last from three to five years, and program progression is organized around "Learning the Business," "Independently Applying Skills and Knowledge," and "Demonstrating Leadership and Influence Skills."
4. Participants receive quarterly evaluations and leaders and sponsors meet at least annually in rater-reliability sessions to review all participants' performance and progress. These sessions are designed to create consistency in the evaluation and mentoring process, among leaders and sponsors.
5. Participants complete four "merit badge" assignments, over and above their day-to-day position responsibilities. The assignments test their creativity and ability to move the metric needle by solving a revenue cycle, patient experience, financial and academic/university business process problem.

Return on the investment:

1. Nine individuals have successfully matriculated through the program since its inception, and all nine hold senior manager or top-tier administrator roles within Emory's physician management, ambulatory services, business services or development or School of Medicine clinical department

areas. Twenty-five individuals are currently in the program, serving in a variety of management roles, across ten Emory departments or business units.

2. To date, two individuals were asked to leave the program after not meeting their development and productivity goals; four individuals left the program before completing it, for family relocation or professional advancement reasons.

3. Emory's business environment has experienced high growth as the academic and health system expands to reach new patient markets. The supply of ready-to-serve MDP graduates has not fully met the organization's demand for senior leaders. Over the past two years, external searches were required to fill three key administrative roles because supply of fully trained MDP participants was insufficient to meet the demand. But the successful placement of nine graduates negated the need to engage search firms or navigate the risky process of finding and on-boarding external talent.

Emory's commitment to create an ideal patient and family experience and an excellent learning experience in the context of a top-tier academic health care environment takes shape with its investment in the careers of tomorrow's health care administrative leaders. The results are apparent, while the lives and professions of the participants are shaped for service to our organization.

EXERCISES

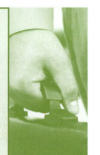

7-1. Get with a partner. This time, select a partner with whom you have not previously worked on the exercises associated with this book. Exchange cover letters and résumés—yes, again. And review with a critical eye toward finding errors. Politely but clearly provide feedback to each other. Get help, in this way, in assuring your cover letter and résumé are error free.

7-2. Select three organizations you believe are the kinds of places you would like to work. Do additional research on them. Answer the following questions: Were they in the news in the last six months? Did they receive any kind of an award in the last 12 months? Was the CEO featured in *Modern Healthcare* or other industry-sector specialized publications? Do not stop at industry-related publications; look for recognition or features in consulting organizations or disease-specific foundations or procedure-related publications. Now play "What do you know about our organization?" with your partner. You ask her "What she knows about your organization?" (One of the three she has selected.) Did she answer the questions above? Reverse procedure.

7-3. Download and connect Skype software for your laptop if you do not already have it. Engage with several partners (three or four) practicing on Skype. Listen to and provide constructive critique, particularly as to eye contact. Remember, you are helping someone improve their skills as you are benefitting from their involvement—so be candid and honest with one another. Practice one-on-one until you are comfortable looking into the camera and speaking. Merge your group with one other. Take turns with three or four people on one end of the call so you can practice with a group. Ask the kind of questions of one another (in role) outlined in the chapter.

Chapter 8

The Interview: Present Your Best Self—And the Finishing Touches

You have come an incredibly long way. You began this journey when you matriculated to college (and again in graduate school). You now stand on the threshold of your professional career. You have put in long, hard hours getting educated in the milieu of health administration. Not only have you learned a great deal about the health care system, its component parts, and theories about how to manage them, but also you have learned a bit about problem solving and critical thinking along the way. Now you are about to take another critically important step: the on-site interview.

At the end of this chapter, you will understand how to prepare for an interview. In addition, the student will understand some of the psycho-social aspects of the interview process, such as wardrobe and body language. Moreover, students will understand and be able to distinguish behavioral interview questions from traditional interview questions and will have some strategies for responding to each. Finally, students will have an understanding of why it is important to raise questions and what questions will be of greatest value in terms of gathering additional information as well as making a positive impression on the prospective employer.

NO, THE RESEARCH IS NOT COMPLETED

In order to reach this part of the process, you have (or should have) researched the prospective employer on the web and beyond. You should have an understanding of some of their organizational strengths and should know about awards and citations they might have received, etc. Furthermore, you should know about ongoing major construction projects or major issues of interest to this organization. That is just to get to this step in the process. Now you want, need, to know more. Search the literature again: *Modern Healthcare*, *The Journal of Medical Practice Management*, *Annals of Long-Term Care*, etc. Take it a step farther this time. Look for articles by key personnel; or perhaps someone from the organization is being interviewed. Perhaps they are being cited for a "best practice." Find the archives of the local newspaper and go back for six months to a year to read about the recent history of the organization. If the organization is a nonprofit, look up their IRS 990 forms. Obtain a copy of their most recent annual report to learn about significant developments in the past year. Be *relentless* in searching out *everything* you can about the organization and be prepared to use it during the interview.

If you are an undergrad going on a job interview, you should have a contact person at this juncture. Schedule a time to talk with them. Before you actually call, think about the questions you might have for that person: What do you want to know about this organization before you go to work there? What do you want to know about this organization before you even have an interview there? Ask about the culture; is it an environment that supports professional growth and development? Get an idea about what the flow of communication is like. Is there a lot of turnover? What does the person with whom you are talking like most about working there? In short, get a picture of how the organization functions operationally to supplement what you have already read and learned about it.

If you are a Master of Health Administration (MHA) student going on an interview for a residency or fellowship, the same sorts of questions apply. In your case, however, call the current resident or fellow and ask them the kinds of questions that appear above. For your part, you will also want to know what the current fellow or resident has been working on during the last 9 or 10 months. You will be there a year or two depending on the type of fellowship; you may want to know (approximately) how many former fellows or residents are still employed by the employer.

In either case, the information you receive from these individuals can be the foundation of more questions when you go for the on-site interview and not just for follow up with the person on the phone. You will make a positive impression, at the on-site interview especially, if you express an awareness of some particular detailed facet of the organization and ask a follow up question of some kind. In other words, use your conversation with your contact person as an educational tool to learn more about the organization. Some of what you learn will help you in the on-site interview. You will be able to reuse some of your first-string questions from the phone conversation in the on-site interview as well, but be certain to have some other questions about the organization in addition to the ones you ask on this phone call. There are some sample questions below in this chapter. You can use these throughout the day of your interview regardless of the title of the person you are visiting with at any point in time, for the committee when they meet as a whole or over dinner or lunch.

CONFIDENCE AND APPEARANCE

Before you even leave your home, be certain you are in crisp attire—cleaned, pressed, and professional from head to toe. You are a professional. Focus on conveying just that attitude.

Be early. Do not be *on time*. Do not, under any circumstances short of your own demise, be late. Arriving 10 to 15 minutes early will allow time for you to gather your thoughts. Use the restroom; primp if you need to straighten up a few things. Get that done and out of the way first when you arrive. Otherwise, use that time to think about what you want to convey; that you are professional; that you are up to the task whatever it may be; and that you are interested in the organization and the people who represent it. *Turn off your cell phone or put it on airplane status. This should NEVER ring while you are interviewing.*

When you meet the first person upon your arrival, be sure to hold your posture upright; smile—show some energy; breathe (deeply—before you actually meet); have a good, firm handshake; make eye contact; lean in just a bit; and let your facial expression reflect recognition of the other person.

There is a great deal going on about now. In the first seven seconds, the person you are meeting with is evaluating you based on your body language, your demeanor, your mannerisms, and the way you are dressed (Goman, 2011). Use this time constructively. It is all pretty subtle, so keep that positive mental image of you as a professional firmly planted in your mind.

Ms. Jones now invites you to have a seat in either her office or the conference room. What do you do? How you sit will also add to the impression of whether you are a good candidate. Let the interviewer direct you to a chair. When you sit down in the chair, do the following:

1. Feel good about yourself and how you look; because you went the extra mile in making sure your appearance was professional, now is a good time to remind yourself of that and let yourself feel good about how you look.

2. Place your feet squarely on the floor. Do not cross your legs. Do not get comfortable. Having your feet on the floor will help you breathe more easily and will not create any distractions such as wiggling your foot incessantly when your legs are crossed.

3. Sit up straight and sit still. You do not want to appear nervous, which is what the body is saying when it moves a lot.

4. Place your hands on your knees. Yes, talk with your hands when appropriate, but for now leave them still in your lap or on your knees.

5. Lean forward toward the interviewer just a bit. This demonstrates serious interest in the position and the interview.

6. Avoid folding your arms. This makes you seem unfriendly or otherwise closed. This is certainly not the time to be either.

7. If you have a habit of playing with your hair, biting your nails, cracking your knuckles, or some other form of nervous habit do not do it here. All of these tic-like behaviors are distracting.

8. Keep your hands out of your pockets. This looks, depending on your perspective, too casual or messy.

9. While you should lean forward just a bit to demonstrate interest, do not invade the interviewer's social space. Keep yourself—all parts of yourself—on your side of the desk or the table. Invading the space of another is irritating to the person whose space is invaded. No reason to alienate anyone at the moment.

10. Use a prop if it helps you look and feel more comfortable. For example, keep a pen poised between your thumb and palm if it helps. Or keep a pen or pencil propped between your thumb, forefinger, and index finger. Do not make it the centerpiece of a fist, however. And do not use it as a drumstick on the table or desk top.

11. Do not stare. Eye contact is a very good thing; staring is a bit freaky. You want to connect with the interviewer by making good eye contact when responding to a question; you do not need to stare them down or let them think you are a member of the living dead (Giang, 2012).

If you do these things you will be off to a running start. When you get to the questions, you will need to give good, cogent, brief (but descriptive) responses.

You should also have a leather or faux-leather folio with you. Again, avoid the froufrou colors and designs in favor of black or brown, something that matches your most common leather accessories. The folio can be zippered or not and should contain an 8 and ½ by 11 pad with a pocket on the opposite side. In the folio you should have two or three copies of your résumé and some examples of your best work from your classes. Good examples might be a competitor analysis, a business plan, a memo, any kind of class deliverable that shows the high quality work of which you are capable. While these are busy people and you do not want to inundate them with unnecessary additional paper for them to read, leaving a good sample of your work with your résumé could be helpful.

THE QUESTIONS YOU MAY BE ASKED

There are basically two kinds of questions. First are the more traditional "tell me about where you want to be in three to five years" types of questions that focus on *who* you are. Second, questions that tell the interviewer *how* you do things, also called *behavioral questions*, have become increasingly popular in the last several years.

"Traditional" Questions

Below is a list of some of the traditional questions you may be asked (some of these are identical to the earlier questions regarding telephone and Skype interviews). You should review these and develop a brief strategy to answer each one of them.

1. Tell me about yourself.
2. What can you offer us?
3. What are your strengths?
4. What are your limitations?
5. Why are you interested in health care administration?
6. What are your ambitions for the future?
7. What do you know about our organization?
8. Why do you want to work for us?
9. What do you find most attractive about the position we are discussing? What is the least attractive?
10. What do you look for in this job?
11. What important trends do you see coming in health care?
12. Describe what you feel would be an ideal working environment.
13. Which do you like better: working with data or numbers, people, things, or words? And why?
14. What other opportunities are you considering?
15. How would you describe your personality?
16. If you could change one thing about your personality at the snap of your fingers, what would it be?
17. How would other people describe you?
18. What are your long-range career goals?
19. Where do you see yourself in three to five years?
20. What has been your biggest mistake?
21. What has been your most significant accomplishment?
22. How do you generally handle conflict?
23. What characteristics make a successful manager?
24. How do you deal with unpleasant or difficult people?
25. Is there anything else about you I should know?

Once again, there is a limitation on how much your faculty, your friends, this book, or anyone else, can do for you. The answers to these questions can only come from you. The challenge to you is that you should have a strategy, the outline of an answer, planted in your head for each and every one of these questions. Most of these can be answered by referring back to the exercises in Chapter 1. How did you respond to those questions? If you really focused and did the exercises in Chapter 1, then many of the answers to the questions listed here will come to you fairly easily. Questions 11, 14, and 20 through 24 are obvious exceptions. But you should be able to answer question 11 based on your recent academic work. The others are all rooted in your own life experience and you merely need to reflect on them and your memory to consider an appropriate response. Short of that, there is not much anyone can do to help you find the answers to these questions. Style of answers will be discussed in more depth below.

Behavioral Questions

Behavioral questions focus not so much on *who are you*, but rather are intended to reveal *how* you do things; how you function in certain situations. Again, you should have a strategy for each of these questions. In the case of behavioral interview questions, your answer should be in the form of a story; have a couple of examples in mind for each question, as these may arise more than once (i.e., examples from work experiences, classroom/group projects, team activities and some non-health care-related experiences).

1. Describe a situation in which you had to lead a project or group of people. What methods did you use that were successful?
2. Describe a problem that you have faced, which had potential impact on other people, or had consequences beyond your responsibility. What decisions did you make and why?
3. Tell me about an assignment you have worked on in the past that did not turn out the way you hoped it would. What did you learn from it?
4. Describe a previous experience when a breakdown in communication caused a major problem. How did you correct it?
5. Give me an example of something you have done that shows initiative.
6. Give me an example of a time you successfully worked within a team.

7. Tell me about a time when someone on your team was not doing their share of the work. How did you handle it?
8. Give me an example of a situation in which you solved a very complex problem. How did you approach it?
9. Tell me about a time when you motivated someone else to take an action or complete a task.
10. Tell me about the time you felt most proud about having completed an assignment or successfully solved a problem.

Here, again, the only person who can answer these questions is you. You might refer to the exercises in Chapter 1 to refresh your identity just a bit; however, even those exercises are of nominal value here because these questions are about *how* you handled various scenarios of life's journey, not so much about *who* you are. In this case, you should examine the list of questions here closely. Reflect back when you have had experiences referenced in the question. Look to the several projects you have worked on during your academic career. There was always someone who was playing the role of social loafer—how did you handle that person? Think about an episode from other aspects of your life. Has there ever been a communications breakdown at the place where you work—or someplace where you worked in the past? Were you ever on a sports team—intramural, club, or varsity—where you were a motivator for your team? Think deeply about the situations referenced by the questions.

When the interviewer is asking behavioral questions, the answers do not necessarily need to come from work or academic-related experiences, especially if you are an undergraduate looking for your first job. Consider the breadth of your experiences and respond to the question using your entire life experience as the prism. For MHA students, it is a little bit different, but not that much. For the MHAs, you will likely have a plethora of group projects on which you worked in your program. These all become good foundations for responding to questions like these. Likewise, however, for both MHAs and undergrads it is perfectly acceptable to

draw from life experiences in work, in volunteer activity, or in some non-health administration related activity so long as it is relevant to answering the question of *how* you did whatever the question seeks to answer.

Notice especially that six of the ten questions deal with some kind of team, communications in a group, or impact on other people. Managing relationships is critically important in management and leadership. Being able to rely on others to accomplish team goals is a necessity. More of a necessity is that others can rely on you.

Who Is Asking Anyway?

Be not surprised by anything regarding how the interview unfolds. The chances are pretty good this will not be a one person sitting down with you for one hour. Depending on the position and the level, this may be a *rotation* where the candidate goes from one office to the next for a half-day or perhaps a full day, or it could be a *panel* interview where a number of people gather in a conference room to (seemingly) grill the candidate for an hour or two, or it could be some combination of the first two. In the case of an administrative fellowship or residency, it most likely will begin with dinner the evening before, followed by a day long set of interviews that are done both individually and in panels. Students will need to be prepared for both the intimate settings of a one-on-one interview in an executive office as well as confronting a panel of 10 to 15 in a conference room. Remember, this is health care, so it is process laden and intended to engage multiple stakeholders.

Answering the Questions with Style

While no one can help you with the substance of how you respond to any of these questions, there are some universal approaches that will benefit you stylistically. How you respond to a question can be as important as the substance you convey. Follow some of these suggestions to improve on the style points behind the substance of your answers.

1. If possible, tell a story. This is much more plausible with behavioral question than traditional ones. Stories are things that people remember. Stories make the content more interesting because they are—or at least, can be—entertaining. Try to have multiple stories for each of the behavioral questions above.

2. Do not ramble. There is a difference between telling a story and retelling your life history. Be careful not to go on and on and on. Tell the story; get to the point. Verbally underscore how this is responsive to the question and then stop.

3. Pause and think. It is good to stop for a moment and consider the answer you are about to give. Think logically; how does A go with B and so forth. Have—and demonstrate—a logical thought process.

4. Have an idea about how what you did (behavioral) or who you are (traditional) would fit into this organization. Can you see yourself succeeding in this role? Can you apply the story (behavioral) or the response to the traditional question to the role at hand and how you might see yourself in that role?

5. A special note about discussing mistakes of the past; if you are confronted with the question "What is the biggest mistake you ever made?" or "Tell me about a project that did not pan out as you expected," do not dwell on how others on the team did not do their share or how you were unfairly treated by the supervisor, or other kinds of complaints about what others did not do or how you were treated unfairly. There are two key words here: Take responsibility. If you made a mistake, or something for which you were responsible did not work, own it, rather than focus on how unfair it may all have seemed. Talk about what went wrong, why and what you learned from it. Indeed, spend the majority of the time it takes to answer focused on the lessons you learned. Employers do not expect people to be absolutely perfect. They do, however, value employees who can take responsibility and also those who learn from mistakes. If you answer this question with a whine about a lazy team member, a crazy faculty member, or an unreasonable supervisor, you will not be considered further. Period.

The interviewer may have a number of things going through their head when they are talking to you. Basically, however, the interviewer is looking for just a few things. First, is the candidate likable? No one wants to be around some kind of self-important, know-it-all, ego maniac. Ick! The interviewer is thinking "We are going to be spending a LOT of time together and I don't need (another?) self-appointed expert who thinks he has all the answers." (Or perhaps you saw the movie *Internship* in which the same question got asked this way: "Would you want to spend an eight-hour layover with this person?") Second, and this is somewhat tied to the first, the interviewer wants someone who will fit in with the culture of the organization. If the organization values high-energy exchanges of ideas and is open, transparent, and debates initiatives, the shy proverbial wallflower may not mix so well with colleagues. Third, the interviewer is looking for value; what kinds of competencies and skills will you bring to the organization and are those going to be worth the salary they are going to pay you? To be abundantly clear, the patients are valuable from a business perspective because they represent revenue. You, on the other hand, are an expense. All good organizations try to maximize revenue and minimize expense. Therefore, you want to be in a position to represent that the expense the organization will incur in bringing you on board is worth the money. Finally, and most certainly not least, the interviewer is looking for people of good character—people who have integrity. No one wants someone in the mix who will jeopardize the good name of the organization by tweeting some celebrity's private health information, or who would falsify records, or steal drugs, and commit other ethical (and legal) violations. Health care organizations rely heavily on their reputations in the communities they serve and not one of them has room for a cheater. There is too much at stake; the patients trust them to provide good care. Competency is but one part of trust. The other part is honesty (Covey, 1989).

IF YOU GET INVITED TO AN INTERVIEW LUNCH, DON'T ORDER THE SPARE RIBS . . .

Frequently a part of the interview process is a meal, either a lunch or a dinner; sometimes it is both. The student will need to know their way around the table to pass this particular test—and, yes, this is a part of the test. About now, you are thinking, "Is he kidding? If there is one thing I know, it is how to eat! I have been doing it forever!" I realize that, but there are some basic rules of etiquette and some subtle hints about eating in a group setting that you might find helpful. If you follow a few basic rules, everyone at the table will appreciate it. Well, let me put it this way: They may not notice you eating, which is a very good thing. Eating is one of those things where you really do not want to be noticed. Nothing good can come from being noticed while eating.

That is the purpose of this section.

BEFORE YOU SIT DOWN

There are a couple of basic things that you should be aware of or do before you even sit down for the meal. Of course, you already look great because you prepared for this part of the interview. Now might be a good time, however, to visit the rest room to "freshen up" your appearance. Do all the little things that go into making a terrific impression: straighten the tie; primp the hair, etc. Second, when approaching the table, watch for seating cues from the host. She may have a specific seat for you in mind or there may be place cards. Be aware! Be certain you have met everyone who will be in the lunch or dinner party. Introduce yourself; shake hands (or not—if that is the custom). Turn off your cell phone or at the very least, put it on airplane setting. This is a job interview. What could be more important that you would want to be interrupted to take a phone call?

LUNCH

The title of the section is not entirely a joke. If you are in a situation, be it lunch or dinner, where you have the opportunity to order from a menu, *do not* order anything that requires the use of your fingers to eat.

This means avoid the ribs, fried chicken, wraps, and sandwiches. All of these, to a greater or lesser degree, end up on your fingers and hands. The sauce from the ribs and grease from the chicken can find its way to your face—which is exactly opposite the image you want to project for an interview. Wraps are notorious for falling apart in your hands and sandwiches have the possibility of doing the same. You are probably in a strange restaurant and may think you are ordering an average ham and cheese sandwich. Then out comes the local interpretation of *The Dagwood* and you have no idea how you will get your mouth around that four-layer, five-inch sandwich. The best way to handle all of this is to avoid ordering anything that might be "hard" to eat.

If you are at lunch, order a salad or soup and salad. It is a healthy lunch and minimizes the opportunity that you will end up wearing the food. OK, the soup can be problematic, so I will address some soup eating tips below. You can either follow those or avoid the soup and stick with the salad by itself, which is probably the better bet.

Remember, this meal is not about the food; it is about the conversation. Do not order the most expensive item on the menu, you will look like you are trying to gouge your host while traveling and eating on their dime. No need to order the least expensive thing either unless it is something you really want. As to the beverage, stay with water, tea, or a soft drink. In the strongest possible terms, this is *not* a meal with which you should be consuming alcohol. Generally speaking, I always suggest that students follow the host's lead on most things at a meal like this one. There can always be one exception, however, and that is the consumption of alcohol. Perhaps your host can operate on the dulled senses associated with a glass of wine or beer at lunch (and, yes, even one glass of either will dull one's senses), but you need to be on your "A" game; you need to be in complete command of your wits. Stay away from booze in all forms. If the would-be boss asks, "Are you sure?" or something like that, just say politely "I am, thank you." Besides, this could be a test question. Perhaps they want to make sure you are not the have-a-drink at lunch kind of person.

With respect to other matters of appearance, for the gentlemen in particular, do not remove your jackets to sit down for lunch. There are two reasons for this: First, I think it simply lacks elegance when a gentleman removes his suit jacket to have lunch. Do you expect to splash around in the food so much that it will soil your jacket? What is the point? Second, if the host retains his (or her) jacket will this not look a bit odd? If he does remove his or her jacket, then you may follow his (or her) lead. I once had a lunch interview in an executive's office and she apologized because she did not have an opportunity to put her suit jacket back on before I was shown in to her quarters. As she was clearly cognizant of the disparity, I said, "That is

perfectly all right" and removed my blazer so we would be on "equal terms" with respect to wardrobe as we dined. I think she appreciated that (and, yes, I was offered the position). Follow the lead of the host. If he or she removes their jacket, then by all means do what you can to make them comfortable by following their lead. If they do not, then yours should remain in place.

DINNER

Dinner is a bit more complicated. Mostly it is more complicated because there are frequently more people involved and there are usually more forks and knives at the table. If you have not seen this many forks, knives, plates, and glasses before, be neither intimidated nor dismayed because I am about to explain this to you and it is not nearly so complicated as it may seem. See Figure 8-1. The next several paragraphs use Figure 8-1 as a reference point.

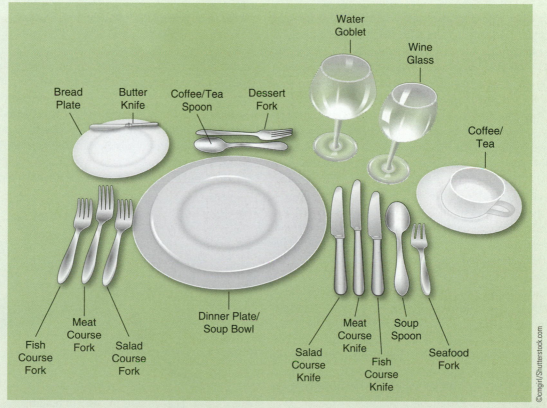

Figure 8-1 A typical banquet place setting.

(continues)

(continued)

There are a few general rules to begin. For the most part, as you go through the various courses of the dinner, you will work *from the outside in* with repect to using the various elements of silverware. Thus, when the soup is served (first), you will use the soup spoon first. When the salad arrives, you will use the salad fork and so forth. By the way, at this point you may not know if you will be getting ice cream or cake (or pie) for dessert because those are dessert implements at the top of the dinner plate. So avoid using those until dessert arrives! Now for a few specifics.

The Napkin. "Wait a minute," you think. "I *know* to put a napkin in my lap, *dude*." Of course you do, but here are some additional helpful hints. When you remove the napkin from its place, which is the first thing you should do when you are seated, fold it in half. By doing this, you will have a clean side for clothes and one to use. If the one you use becomes soiled, you can easily refold by and retain one clean side for your clothes and one to use. If this happens again, you can refold again. You may need to place a soiled side down on your lap, but at least you will have a clean side up. If you end up using (soiling) all four sides of the napkin, you may want to revisit your eating habits.

You can also use your napkin to communicate. If you must leave the table during the course of the meal, after saying the requisite "excuse me" to all concerned, you place the napkin on the seat of your chair. This says "I am going to return" to the wait staff. While you are gone the staff may refold your napkin, or they might even replace it, or they may do nothing, but at least you have told them you will be returning. When you leave the napkin on the table at your place setting, that says "I am done and am leaving."

Soup and the Soup Spoon. If the soup is too hot you should (a) put an ice cube from your water glass in it; (b) blow on it; (c) blow on it after you put the ice cube in it; or (d) do nothing. If you answered "d" you were correct. In fact, this applies to any food that may be too hot, but all too often the soup is guilty of this and it comes out first, so I mention it here. Just wait for a minute or two and it will cool down. When you do eat it, skim the surface of the soup with the spoon using a motion away from your body. Hold the spoon like you do a fork. See

Figure 8-2. Fill the spoon to about $\frac{1}{2}$ or $\frac{2}{3}$ full, then slowly and carefully lift the spoon and its contents to your mouth. This is the proper way to eat soup. Do not fill the spoon. Skim or scoop away from you. Bring the spoon slowly upward. Do not bend over so your face is right on top of the soup dish; do not slurp from the spoon; do not hold the spoon like a shovel; do not pick up the bowl and drink from it directly.

Bread and Butter: Notice the placement of the bread and butter plate on the upper left of the diagram. This is always the proper placement. When you receive the bread basket, take a piece and place it on this plate. Likewise the butter, use this knife to take some of the butter and put in *on this plate.* Do not take the butter from the main butter dish and butter your bread. Take just enough to use with the piece of bread and put it on the bread plate. When eating the bread, break off a piece *first*, butter it, and then eat it. Do not butter the bread, then bite into it, rebutter, etc. Ewww.

What is with all those glasses? Well, this is a banquet setting, so there is a white wine glass, farthest to the right, a red wine glass, and a water goblet. At a full banquet, you might be asked which wine you would like, you respond, and the other glass would be removed. At an interview meal you probably will not see all of these glasses. In any event, at an interview meal, the smart job candidate stays with water or requests iced tea or a soft drink. If for some reason you feel you absolutely must have an alcoholic

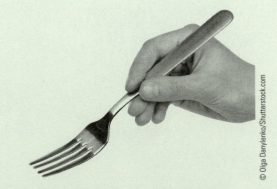

Figure 8-2 The "American" way of holding a fork—this is proper.

beverage, remember the rule from the reception: "One and done."

The salad. You notice the diagram has both a salad fork and a salad knife. Sometimes the salad has chunks of tomato or wedges of lettuce or egg halves that simply cannot, or should not, be eaten in one bite. Rather than poke that baby with a fork and hold up there for a two or three bite sub-serving, use the knife to reduce it to a bite-sized piece.

The entrée. The rules for handling this are pretty much the same as the salad. There will be a meat or seafood entrée (unless you are a vegitarian or vegan and have asked your host to make arrangements for you in advance) along with a starch and a vegetable. Again, use the knife to cut the serving for a bite the size that makes sense for your mouth. If you want to savor the flavor of two items at the same time, put them both on your fork in delicate amounts that permit easy access to your pie hole so you do not over stuff your face. Do not, *ever*, have one thing in your mouth and then put another on your fork then open your mouth to put the second item in. Ewwwww. Really. No one; *no one* wants to see that.

The dessert. The same general rules follow here, except there are no knives. Usually your fork or spoon will be sufficient to slice or scoop whatever needs to be sliced or scooped. Just keep the amounts on your spoon or fork to a reasonable size. Perhaps there should be one additional guideline here: no seconds. Again, you want to appear moderate and reasonable, not gluttonous.

How to hold the implements. You will recall in the discussion about soup a reference to the Figure 8-2 on how to hold a fork. Figure 8-2 shows the proper way to hold a fork while dining. Figure 8-3 shows exactly how *not* to hold a fork while dining. You are not applying for a job that involves digging in any form, so there is little need to hold your fork in a way that resembles a shovel. If you hold your fork (or spoon) in a fashion that looks like this, relearn the new grip in Figure 8-2 and practice.

In terms of using the knife and fork for cutting, the grip on the fork is slightly different. You will need to change the grip to get better leverage, so follow the example in Figure 8-4. That way you can get sufficient leverage to hold the item in place, which is the way you want to use the fork, so the knife can do its job in making the cut.

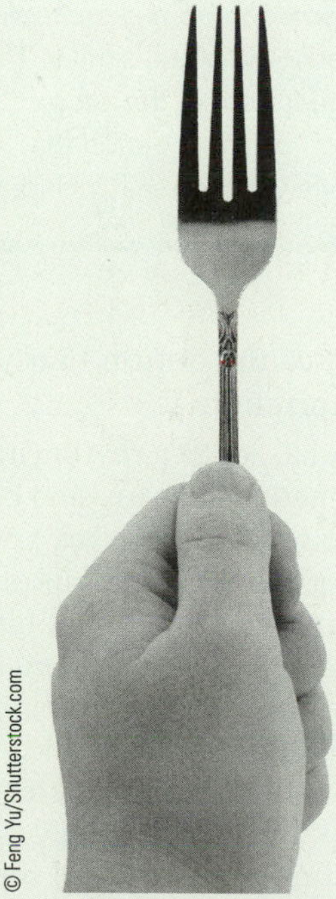

Figure 8-3 The "shovel" grip of the fork—this is inappropriate.

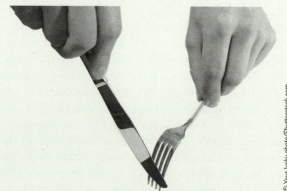

Figure 8-4 Proper way to hold a knife and fork while cutting.

(*continues*)

(continued)

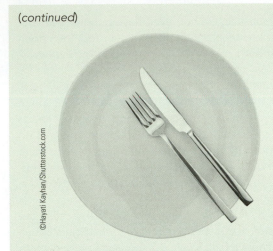

©Hayati Kayhan/Shutterstock.com

Figure 8-5 Proper placement for utensils when you have finished eating.

When you are done eating, you do not just leave the implements just any old way, as these too can be used to communicate. To say "I am done eating," put the knife and the fork pointing inward toward the plate from the 4 o'clock position on the clock face as shown in Figure 8-5. Remember, then you can put the napkin on the table next to the place setting, on the left, to join in telling the wait staff that you are done.

BEFORE YOU LEAVE

Be certain to appropriately say farewell to everyone at the table. If there are people there who are part of the interview team whom you will not see again in the process, be certain to get their business cards as you will want to write them a thank you note later. Be certain you thank the host. It does not matter that "the company is paying for it." The resources came from someone's budget and someone decided to invest in this way. It could be the host; it may be someone else. You may never know. So thank the host for the meal and the conversation.

There are, of course, many nuances to this process. The custom of manners dates back many centuries. Manners exist for good reasons, not the least of which include facilitating the flow of good relationships and commerce. You may want to explore if your student club could ask if your campus career services office could put together an "etiquette dinner" at which a speaker trained in the art of etiquette could provide your group with more detail than is possible here. Or perhaps your student group could arrange for someone from campus dining services, a local restaurant or some place similar. This is certainly not an exhaustive treatment of the subject, but hopefully provides you enough of a foundation that you have confidence in any interview setting that includes a meal.

HOW CURIOUS ARE YOU?

Interviewers all have their own techniques for evaluating candidates. While the four basic elements discussed above are pertinent characteristics, the interviewer probably is looking beyond merely the answers to the questions to make his determinations. One of the ways you can demonstrate that you will bring value to the organization is to demonstrate that you know something about it and are curious to learn more. This also has the implicit message of saying you think you might like the place, and people mostly reciprocate feelings they feel from others. In other words, curiosity can make you seem likable and at the same time reinforce the notion that you will bring value to the organization.

Every interview has its own rhythm and its own ebb and flow of information transmission back and forth. Somewhere in the process, however, you are going to have an opportunity to ask questions of the organization's representatives. (If you do not have this opportunity, you may want to consider this a red flag. If the organization seems to be a one-way street in the way it communicates in the interview process what do you suspect it would be like working there?) Whether you are an MHA seeking a fellowship or an undergrad looking for that first job, there are some things you might consider asking your prospective employer. Adapt the questions below to suit your purposes.

Questions for MHA Administrative Fellowship/Residency Candidates

1. Is the fellowship project based or rotation based?
2. One or two years?
   a. How does first year differ from second year?
3. How many fellows will you accept for <fill in the year>?
4. Do you enjoy being the only fellow? As part of a group of fellows?
5. Are you lead or support on projects?
6. Is the office for fellows shared or does the fellow have an individual office?
7. Do you host a Fall Preview Day?
8. Who is the preceptor?
9. Describe the relationship with the preceptor(s)?
10. Do you have adequate access to leadership? 1:1? How often? Easy to reach?
11. How highly structured is the fellowship? Do you have an opportunity to be selective in the projects to which you are assigned? How are your assignments determined?
12. Were your expectations clear before beginning fellowship?
13. Have you had the freedom to customize fellowship based on personal preference?
14. What are past fellows doing now? What are their titles? Are they still with the organization?
15. What year was fellowship established?
16. Do hospital employees understand the role of the fellow?
17. Would you want to be hired there?
18. What made you choose this fellowship?
19. How do you position fellowships within the organization?
20. What kind of exposure will I have to senior leadership and governing bodies while I am in this fellowship?

Questions for Both MHA and Undergrad Fellowship/Job Candidates

1. Is the organization for-profit, or not-for-profit?
2. What is the culture of the hospital?
3. Are the administrators teaching focused? Will they help me grow professionally?
4. Are there mentors or are other leaders assigned to coaching or developmental roles?
5. Is this a formal or informal environment? Do you call people by their first names?
6. What are you looking for in this position?
7. Is there any preference given to affiliation through school?
8. What are your future plans?
9. What is the timeline of application process?
10. What is it like to live in <fill in the blank of the city name>?
11. What is the size of the city, size of hospital?
12. How does your organization measure success?
13. What is the next initiative to be put into action from the Strategic Plan? What is the five-year roll-out plan for strategic projects?
14. Will I have access to hospital and system-level executives? Pre-arranged meetings or as needed?
15. Who are your competitors and what efforts are you taking to stay on top of the market?
16. After the first year on the job, how will you know if I am successful? How will I know?
17. What attracted you to the organization?
18. What keeps you here?
19. What ongoing or emerging projects are you most excited about?
20. How transparent are things within this organization? If not, is that something you are moving toward?
21. How will you describe your organization in five years? What are the primary differences from today?
22. What differentiates your organization?
23. What attributes do successful leaders embody in your organization?
24. What kinds of advancement opportunities have you seen for previous fellows/employees with similar education and experience?

These are only general suggestions. These will be much more powerful if you tailor them to the specific organization or unit in which you are being considered. Questions about the competitors or the city can certainly be augmented with some specific material. For example, if you are interviewing at East Cupcake Memorial Hospital that has ranked in the Top 100 hospitals for cardiac care, you might ask if West Cupcake is making competitive inroads. Or if the shoe is on the other foot and you are interviewing at West Cupcake, take note of the stature of East Cupcake and ask what the West Cupcake strategy is for dealing with the situation. Your prior research about the organization may answer a number of these questions. To the extent it does not, it may help you tailor the question to the specific circumstances for the organization where you are interviewing.

Usually, at the close of the interview, the interviewer will say something like "Is there anything else you would like to tell me" or words to that effect. Here is where you should have a strong closing statement. You will need to be able to think on your feet a bit for this one because you will want to incorporate some of what you have discussed during the interview in these comments. Certainly, you want to express your appreciation for being considered and for the interviewers' time. Comment on how interesting it was to learn more about their organization. If there was something new you learned and were impressed by it, mention that. If you think the job would challenge you in ways that would give you an opportunity to grow, mention that. At this moment, you should be expressing confidence that you can do the job; look your interviewer in the eye and relate to them that you found the time with them interesting and educational. This does not need to be a long-winded speech, just a 30- to 60-second statement.

If your interest in the position has strengthened as a result of the interview experience, then say so. If it has not, then offering a professional "I remain interested" is appropriate. (There is no point in burning a bridge here. Depending on how the rest of your job search goes, you may be more interested in this than you think.) Unless you found that the interview experience just wanted to make you hurl, there is no need for something like "You are kidding, right?

You expect me to take this job?!" Even if you did want to hurl, it would not be professional to express your lack of interest in the job in that particular fashion.

In any event, do not make any rash decisions at this point. The decision point on whether or not you would accept the job is still down the road, and you need to give it the careful consideration it deserves.

Make Your Own Observations and Assessment

The questions above are intended to serve as a guide and not an absolute. You should fashion them to fit your own situation. If you are talking on the phone with a contact in the organization and you merely read these, it will sound—well, like you are reading them. Do not! Use them as conversation starters or conversation fillers; do not memorize them or use them as if from a script.

Regardless of whether you use any of these questions or your own or some permutation of both, the purpose in asking is not to make you sound smart or even to create the impression that you did your homework on the organization. The other reason not to memorize the questions is so you can focus on the answer; not trying to remember the next question. You ask these—and other—questions to elicit information. So what do you do with the answers? Presumably, you asked so you could learn. Now that you have learned, you do not want to forget. As discussed previously, you could be managing several potential opportunities, so you need to keep track of your impressions and of material facts you have learned in the process.

During the interview, of course, you want to enjoy the interplay and participate in the exchange of information. Be in the moment and engage fully in the process. But having asked questions and learned a good bit about the organization, you will want to preserve that information to compare with other potential employers. So when the interview is over—*not* while it is occurring—whip out your iPad or laptop or whatever portable device you have and start tapping. Enter all the notes you can remember from the meetings.

What did you think of the interviewer? Was he or she likable to you? Did you see them as competent? Did they appear to be warm like a good coach or teacher? Or did they seem a bit aloof and distant? Did you feel as though you were being recruited? Or did you feel like a piece of meat on a slab being examined before purchase? OK, that last one is a bit extreme. But the point is that you should feel as though you are in a two-way conversation; that the environment, as projected through the interviewer(s) and interview process, is one in which you can grow and thrive.

In addition to your observations about the interviewer what are your impressions of the organization? Is it profitable and stable financially? Equally, perhaps more, importantly, how were you treated? Did you meet more than one or two people? When you asked questions of your hosts, did they seem transparent? Were they candid? What did the culture seem like with regard to work-life balance? Did anyone slip you a business card and say "call me so we can talk off-line about this place"? (This is a *huge* red flag.) Did you like the people you met? (This is often something that is reciprocated; in other words, if you felt good about the meeting, chances are better than even that they did also.) By itself, this is not determinative. After all, some people like Homer Simpson, but they probably would not hire him.

Visualize working with the people you met. Visualize getting up early in the morning and spending the entire day with those people. Consider what they want the person in this position to do. Do the skills you have match the potential employer's expectations? Can you do the job? Do you want to do it with the people you just met?

The bottom line: Would you take the job if it were offered?

Time to Sit Back and Wait for "The Call"

Not so much.

First, make certain you have the name, title, and mailing address for everyone you met during the interview. If you do not have this information, get in touch with your contact person and ask for it.

Second, send a handwritten thank you note to everyone who was a part of the interview process. Everyone. Each one of those people gave up a part of their day to meet or be with you. Chances are some will need to come in a bit early or stay a bit late to catch up on the work they could have gotten done while meeting with you, so expressing some appreciation to them for their time would be appropriate. Again, a handwritten note will receive a measure of attention that an e-mail will not. This will help your chances. By itself, no, this is not determinative. But taken as part of the overall package you represent, it is another positive.

But there is more. Where are you with the other prospective interviews? Have you sent a thank you note for the phone interview with the other organizations? Do you need to do more research on some other prospect? Do you need to contact your references to make sure you are keeping them informed on your progress? Or do you need to let them know that someone may be calling them?

There is one more thing. Because this is all likely taking place during the latter part of your academic career, the faculty sure would appreciate it if you would turn in some homework and show up for class.

EVALUATING THE OFFER AND SALARY NEGOTIATION

It is most likely this will not be much of a negotiation at this level as it will become for you in, say, 5 or 10 years. Generally, large organizations (even small hospitals) have fairly rigid scales of compensation they will pay for incoming personnel. This applies to both the undergrads seeking their first job as well as to the MHA seeking the fellowship/residency (and to MHAs looking for their first job, as well). There are a few things you can look for, however, and perhaps impact the outcome around the margin somewhat.

Wage scales will vary geographically. The position that goes for $45,000 in San Antonio probably commands $85,000 in New York City. The relative cost of living in various geographic areas drives what employers can and will pay, at least in part. Thankfully, this is one place where the web can help you get prepared for the differences. Google "cost of living comparison" and pick the calculator you like the best. These can get you somewhat acclimated to the new environment if you happen to be moving to a new location. If you intend to move to a new location, part of your interview preparation should include this comparison. Sometimes, for the individual moving to a new location, organizations will pay moving expenses. This is more typical at the upper echelon; however, sometimes MHAs entering into residencies will receive a stipend that will cover at least part of the cost of relocating.

Another question about salary is when to discuss it. You should not raise this topic at the interview. If the prospective employer opens this line of conversation, that is their prerogative (more on that below). It is, however, unseemly for the candidate to ask at the interview "How much does this pay?" It casts the candidate in the light of being focused more on the money and less on the work. It is a real downer for the employer. The interview should be about the position at hand, the people involved, and whether you and the organization agree that you have the skills, knowledge, and abilities to do the job. Salary discussions should be in conjunction with a job offer or a second on-site/final interview. Oftentimes, for entry-level positions, this is not a point of discussion because the salary is announced or otherwise disclosed on the front end of the process. Presumably, you would not go to the time and trouble to apply and interview if you were not interested for reasons related to salary. So this issue falls into one of four buckets:

1. The salary was disclosed as part of the job announcement;
2. The salary was not disclosed and was not mentioned by the interviewer (and should not be mentioned by the candidate) during the interview;

3. The salary was not disclosed and the subject was broached by the interviewer during the interview; and
4. The salary was disclosed after the interview as part of the job offer.

Items one and two have been addressed above. The discussion below will focus on situations three and four.

If the subject of compensation arises at the interview, it will most likely come in one of two forms. The interviewer says:

1. "The position pays, 'x,' would you remain interested in the job with a salary at that level?" (Or words to that effect.)
2. "Do you have a salary in mind?" or "What are your salary requirements?"

In the first instance, your research should have led you to some notion of what the job would pay. This is where talking to people who work in the organization pays off. If you have done your homework and understand what the compensation has been in the past for this job, then you can pretty easily answer the question. If you have not been able to uncover this information in your research, or you are unsure for other reasons, you can respond with something like "Yes, I believe so; however, I would like to visit with your HR department to discuss other aspects of the total compensation package." This defuses a potentially awkward situation. Candidly, this might be the best response even if you do know what to expect and the offer is in the range you expected it would be. The reason you want to push this discussion outside of the interview process is twofold: (1) you do not want the organization using your salary preference as a disqualifier and (2) there are other factors that go into evaluating the total offer.

The second question above borders on unfair at this level. This, too, is a question you need to politely deflect because you do not want salary to be a disqualifier. Frankly, the organization already should have a sense of the value of the position. For that reason, this question is an effort to see if they can save a buck. If they are prepared to pay $50,000 and your answer is that you were expecting to make $45,000, guess what? You may have just given away $5,000 in salary. Your response to this question should be something like "Obviously, I would like to do well, but I expect you have a better idea than I do about the value of the position."

The salary by itself is not the only issue. What are the fringe benefits like? What kind of health insurance does the organization provide? What is your share of its cost? How much does the organization provide to match your contribution to retirement? (Yes, you should be thinking of this at your age. Or do you intend to work until you are 80? Or until you die? More on this later.) Will you have to pay for parking? How are vacation and sick leave accrued? The discussion of these questions is why this should not be a part of the interview process. These kinds of discussions are best held with an expert from HR; variations in them could be important. Let us say, for example, that you were expecting a $50,000 salary, but the offer is $45,000. The complete picture, however, is that your health insurance costs will be a measly $50 per month, with copays of $5 for a physician visit and $5 for prescription drugs. (In case you do not realize it, this is an incredibly generous package.) On top of that, the organization making the offer will provide up to $7,000 in relocation expenses, has free parking, contributes 6% above and beyond the amount of your salary in a retirement plan and gives you four weeks of vacation in the first and all ensuing years. Compare this to another hypothetical offer of $55,000 in which there are no relocation expenses, an insurance plan that costs $100 a month with $10 copays for seeing the doc and a 25% copay for prescription drugs, charges $30 a month for parking, contributes 4.5% above and beyond the amount of your salary into a retirement account and provides only two weeks of vacation for the first two years, allowing you to earn an additional week in each of years three and four. Which is the better offer? This is just the financial part of the equation. You need to factor in that subjective "how do I feel about working with these people and will I have a

chance to grow into greater responsibilities" perspective. Giving yourself an opportunity to reflect on these issues is precisely why you do not want to say "yes, I want to start tomorrow" or "No, you must be crazy" impulsively on the spot.

The value of the retirement contribution and health insurance deserves special attention. You may be tempted to think that retirement and health insurance do not matter much. While at the age of 24, 25, 26—under 30 for the most part—you do not get sick much and are in mostly low risk categories for premature health issues (unless you behave so badly as to increase your risk by smoking, drinking and driving, using recreational drugs, using firearms or some combination of the foregoing, etc.). Right now you think you are going to live forever, so who needs health insurance, right? Do not engage in such a delusion. Health insurance is a major benefit and if you picked up on this in your class on risk management, you do not know when you will need to have it. Accident or illness can strike suddenly and without warning; be prepared by being covered. Truly generous health insurance benefits are hard to find, so make certain your prospective employer includes health insurance in the offer and if you have the good fortune to look seriously at more than one job opportunity, take the time to compare how each of your prospective employers structures this benefit.

Likewise, the retirement contribution is important. Again, you may not see it that way because at your age being that old is not only an abstract concept, but generally just a crummy idea. Who wants to be old? Nobody, except those who die young. What will you use to support yourself and your spouse when you are 70 years old? And in case you have not been paying attention, Social Security is in difficult financial straits with a growing number of beneficiaries and a diminishing number of contributors. Do the math. It is much less expensive for you to set up a retirement account NOW than it will be 30 years from now when you are 55 or so, and have coronary stenosis compounded by high blood pressure and arthritis in your left hip. So, compare; evaluate what the employers are contributing to your retirement plan in addition to the deduction you are contributing from your salary.

Finally, compare the vacation and sick leave policies. These are expenses to the employer. To some degree, these policies may reflect the organization's commitment to work-life balance.

If the organization makes you a formal offer after your on-site interview, it will most likely contain not only the base salary, but much of the information just discussed. The same kind of analysis applies: look at the salary, the health insurance, the retirement contribution, the cost of parking, and the vacation and sick leave policies and make certain you are making an apples to apples comparison. If the offer only speaks to salary, be certain to ask about these other important considerations before saying "yes" or "no."

If you have concerns about any one of these things, now is the time to raise the issue. For example, if you are going to relocate over a long distance and the organization has not mentioned relocation expenses as part of its offer, now is the time to let them know that is important. Particularly if you like the opportunity and the other matters are agreeable. If you do not ask, they will not know and the opportunity for both of you may be lost. The most they can say is "we do not provide moving expenses." Then, of course, your next question is whether the compensation might be adjusted a bit so you can recapture that expense over time. If the answer to this, too, is "no," then you may have some thinking to do. If you loved the people and the place while you were there and it is a prestigious place like "Best Hospital West of the Rockies (BHWR)," you may want to go ahead and accept the offer in spite of a more generous offer from East Cupcake. Conversely, East Cupcake may be a terrific place to be because you will get much more exposure to so many different aspects of the profession as it is a smaller place, whereas at BHWR you would be in charge of the postage meter.

It is not all about the salary. It is about whether the job would provide you an opportunity to make a positive impact on an organization, and thus the care received by patients, while further developing your professional skills. The salary and benefits package are things that make it possible for you to live reasonably well and afford you the opportunity to engage in meaningful work in a good place. They are not ends by themselves. It is not about the money alone. It is about serving others and making a positive difference in their lives.

The Ethics of Accepting an Offer

Once having decided, it is your ethical obligation to, as an old saying goes, "stay hitched." One of the reasons it is important for you to try to balance the timing of interviews and offers is to afford yourself the maximum number of opportunities from which to select without violating any duty you might owe to any particular organization. As an applicant—as a professional—you owe each organization to which you apply for a position—whether it is for an internship, fellowship, residency, or a job—the duty of dealing in good faith. This does not mean you need to tell each organization the precise details of the conversations you might be having with the others. It does mean, however, that if you say you are interested that you mean it. It also means that if you say "yes," you mean that, too.

We have said more than once that health care is a small world. Your reputation will travel fast, particularly if it is bad. You can be certain if you stiff somebody on a job offer by saying "yes" and reneging because you found one for an extra $5,000 that will come back to bite you some day. Guaranteed. Karma exists for certain. The person you lied to—yes, that is exactly what it is—will remember you for a long time. Sometime down the road, however, when you see an ad in *Modern Healthcare* for Director of Surgery job that reports to the COO in another organization and you figure now is your time so you apply. Then you discover the COO is the person you lied to eight years ago when you reneged on the fellowship he offered you. Oops.

Of course, getting caught is *not* the reason to avoid this kind of duplicitous behavior. Understanding that you have a simple duty of good faith and fair dealing with your prospective employers should be sufficient. When you receive an offer; review it. If you feel like you need more time to review it, ask for it. If you need to respond then you need to say "yes" or "no." Once you say "yes," then you are obligated to stop interviewing. Period. You are done. If you continue beyond this point, then it will be assumed by others that your acceptance means nothing and that you are interested only in yourself and the best short-term gain you can achieve for yourself. As a consequence, no one should rely on anything you have to say.

CONCLUSION

The focus at the beginning of this chapter was on giving yourself permission to feel good about yourself; about taking pride in your professional appearance. In addition, you read a good deal about how to conduct yourself in the interview and how to interpret body language and project your own. A host of questions that you might confront in the interview were included. Information regarding the traditional questions of *who* you are and behavioral questions focused on the *how* you respond to certain situations was also provided. In addition, some suggested lines of inquiry you might make at the time of the interview were outlined. You were also advised to make notes of your observations so you can later compare the cultures of organizations that (hopefully) will be competing for your affections. OK—competing for your professional engagement.

Beyond how to appear for the interview and manage the questions, you were advised that there are things you can do after the interview to (a) prepare for another interview and (b) express appreciation for the one you just completed. A good bit of discussion regarding salary negotiation and evaluation of offers was presented to enable you to understand how to evaluate employment offers. With the tools from this chapter, the student should understand, and be able to apply, principles about how to handle the interview from arrival on the scene to evaluating the employment offer.

You have done a terrific job of living up to expectations of a young professional so far. The next steps will be what to do when you get there.

THE CASE INTERVIEW: OR HOW TO MESS WITH YOUR HEAD

There is a third type of interview that is sometimes used, but not nearly so often as the behavioral interview or the traditional interview and that is called the case interview. This will primarily have application for MHA students seeking residencies and fellowships, but it would not hurt for undergrads to be familiar with it.

There are three types of case interviews:

1. Business situation: "A hospital has very little revenue and needs to decide between investing in new imaging equipment or updating the cardiac care unit. Which would you choose?"

There is no right answer to this scenario. There is not nearly enough information to make a clear-cut decision regarding the question. So the interviewer is not so interested in you tossing a coin and choosing the imaging equipment if it comes up heads. What they want you to focus on here are: Problem-solving logic; your ability to apply quantitative measures and relationships; and how you understand people and organizations. In part, they want to see how you think in big picture terms.

2. Back of small napkin analysis: "How many public parks are there in the United States?" Again, the answer is not the point. Here the interviewer

(continues)

(*continued*)

is looking for: logical and creative thinking; basic quantitative ability; and comfort with making assumptions. How would you go about crafting a guestimate in response to this question? Would you consider one of the following assumptions to help devise an answer? Do you have any experience or know anything that might help shed some light? At the beginning, you will need to make an assumption. Have a rationale for that assumption. There are three immediately below, not necessarily right or wrong. (Googling for the answer will not help you.)

- *Number of Parks per 100,000 people*
- *Number of Parks per city*
- *Number of Parks per 1000 square miles*

3. Brain teasers: "How many dimes placed on top of each other would it take to reach the top of the Empire State Building?" Again, Google will not help with the answer. What the interviewer is looking for is your ability to generate multiple hypotheses. There is pressure to get to the answer. Can you do so and retain your natural poise. In this case, you might need some particular pieces of information and should ask for them.

- *Height of Empire State Building*
- *Depth of dime*
- *Width of dime*
- *More information—what does "on top of each other" mean?*

In every single case interview question, the organization, through its interviewer is looking for your ability to analyze, in addition to your level of intellectual curiosity. Furthermore, the interviewer is looking for analytical sharpness and creative problem solving along with communication skills, motivation, energy, and stamina.

Interviewers are most certainly not looking for a single right answer. They are not even particularly interested in hearing what you may know about functional or even deep business analysis of their industry. Why this style of interview? In a phrase, the employer seeks to understand your ability to solve problems and how

you think. Are you comfortable with ambiguity? How do you handle quantitative and qualitative analyses? Are you logical in your approach? Can you engage in dialogue about the problem without being overwhelmed or intimidated?

This type of interview is particularly popular with consulting firms. Why? This is what consultants do every day. They approach complex problems with insufficient information. They gather what they need to know, and break down the complex problem to a workable couple of principles. In a very ambiguous environment develop one or more answers to the question.

There are a few key steps to approaching this kind of question. First, summarize the situation. Break down the pieces; think out loud; ask for more information. Try verbalizing and describe different approaches; then pick one. Then focus on what you see as the important issues; be creative; listen to the interviewer; draw on your own experience; reach a conclusion.

Fortunately, you can put the problem into a couple of contexts for thinking about all this material:

a. PCCC: patients, competitors, capabilities, cost. This is almost always useful. Look back at the question regarding the imaging equipment and cardiac unit. How do you go about making that choice: Think about the number of and fashion in which patients will be affected. Consider what the competitors are doing, planning to do or recently have done that is relevant to this question. What are the organization's current capabilities? And, of course, how much will each cost?

b. PSPL: price, service, promotion, location. This is better suited for a marketing related question. Modify the question a bit. "The organization recently purchased a new 128-slice CT machine that is not meeting revenue projections. What do you do?" Then consider each of the elements here, much as the way you did in the preceding paragraph. Are the prices too high? Are the radiologists too slow to get the reports to the referring physician? (This speaks to service—and is a frequent problem in real life, actually.) Have we promoted the device correctly? Sufficiently? Do we have it (correcting this might be a bit impractical) in the best location?

c. Profitability Analysis:
   a) Profits = Revenue − Costs
   b) Revenue = Price × Volume
   c) Costs = Fixed + Variable: good for profit

Taking question 1 above, I modified the question in a slightly different way. "The organization recently purchased a new 128-slice CT machine. It has not proven to be profitable. What do you do?" This is a simple case of applying quantitative analysis. We may need to raise prices or improve volume to increase revenue. We can examine the cost side of the equation, but only in a limited way. The cost of the device is fixed and the monthly payment cannot be changed. We can, however, look at variable costs in an effort to identify potential savings.

You should always feel free to ask for additional information when you think it might be helpful. Do not, however, evidence any frustration when you hear, "We do not have that information." Remember, it is not the answer that counts in this type of question; it is your thought process. Use the frameworks above to help you sort out the information. Draw on your own experiences as well as any factual material you may happen to know. Use analogies to help piece the answer together.

EXERCISES

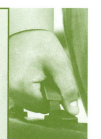

8-1. Make a list of the places you think you would like to work when you graduate. Put them in priority order by whatever prism you are using to determine desirability. For the first three, write down what you know about the organization that makes it attractive to you. List all the reasons you think it would be a good place to work. Now look at those same three organizations and list reasons why one might not want to work there.

8-2. Conduct a mock interview. Get two partners. One will be the interviewer; one will be the observer. You will be interviewed by a partner who will use between 5 and 10 questions from the traditional question list. You should not see or be told the questions in advance. Have the partner ask the questions and give your best response. The observer partner should take notes regarding both the substance and style of your answer, including such things as did you seem nervous or uncertain? Did you look the interviewer in the eye? Did you sit slightly forward, feet on the floor? Upon completion, share an open and honest critique. Now rotate the roles and repeat until all three in the group have been interviewed, been interviewers and been observers.

8-3. Repeat Exercise 8-2 and use only 5 to 10 behavioral questions.

8-4. Evaluate the two job offers in the text. Which one offers the better financial outcome for you? Make assumptions that resemble your own circumstances where there is insufficient information. Include an estimate for your federal tax liability as well as the impact of the fringe benefits.

BIBLIOGRAPHY

Covey, S. (1989). *Seven Habits of Highly Effective People.* New York: Simon & Schuster.

Doyle, A. (2014). *About.com Job Searching*. Retrieved March 12, 2014, from About.com: www.jobsearch.about.com

Giang, V. (2012, May 21). *11 Things Your Interviewer is Thinking During the Interview*. Retrieved May 22, 2012, from Business Insider.com: http://www.BusinessInsider.com

Giang, V. (2012, May 8). *12 Facts About Body Language You Should Know*. Retrieved May 12, 2012, from Business Insider: http://www.BusinessInsider.com

Goman, C. K. (2011, February 3). *Seven Seconds to Make a First Impression*. Retrieved June 27, 2012, from Forbes.com: http://www.forbes.com

Hansen, K. (n.d.). *Managing the Case Job Interview*. Retrieved March 12, 2014, from Quintessential Careers: www.quintcareers.com

Chapter 9

Look Out World! Here I Come: Accepting the Job and Professional Ethics

So now you have nearly completed all the course work, suffered the insufferable, borne the unbearable, and arrived to the point where you need to make a decision. "Do I want to accept the offer I have? Or should I wait and see how the other interview goes next week? If I wait will the job still be there for me? If I do not, am I settling?"

"Can I say 'yes' then change my mind if the other place is better?"

"How do I go about continuing to learn?"

"What's the right thing to do?"

At the end of this chapter, students should have an understanding of professional "fit," the need to meet the challenge of lifelong learning, and a better understanding of ethical behavior as a job candidate.

WHAT IS *GOOD FIT*?

The answer to the question of "fit" relies, in part, on two things. First, how well do you know yourself? Remember the self-awareness exercises we did early in the book? Now is a time to reflect on what you learned as a result of those exercises. Do you need freedom on the job to be creative and effective? Or do you need a more structured environment that provides frequent feedback? Does the organization seem to embrace values with which you are comfortable?

Is the job going to permit you to achieve things in ways that are meaningful to you? Or would you feel overwhelmed on day one?

Again, no professor can answer this in a Power-Point presentation and you surely cannot Google the answer. Looking in the mirror can be uncomfortable, but that is OK. As we said earlier, if you are comfortable, you are not growing. The challenge for you now is to assess what you know about the job and about the organization and measure that against your own values, strengths, weaknesses, needs, and preferences. And that brings us to the second part of this question of fit.

The second part is how well do you know the organization that just made you the offer? Did you do enough research when you were in the job search phase that you know a great deal about them? How did you feel while you were there? Could you see yourself working with the people you meet? Is the job as you understand it something that you *want* to do? Is this a job for which you are competent, but that would also permit you an opportunity to grow as a professional; learn new skills; develop some of your other talents?

This is what it means when you hear that the prospective employer not only needs for you to be a good fit for them, but it also needs to be a good fit for you also. Only a part of this comes from the job description. The other part comes from the culture of the organization. What are the norms with regard to the way people treat one another? What did you see while you were at the on-site interview? Did people acknowledge one another in the hallways? Were there many of people smiling, looking as though they were intently engaged in what they were doing? Did you sense camaraderie or tension in the room? Did the organization's leadership welcome diverse perspectives? Or did the CEO seem to think he had all the answers?

Consider this: During the interview, you are walking down a corridor of a hospital with a vice president and you both see a discarded pen on the floor. What do you learn by watching her response? If she bends over to pick it up and keeps it until she sees a trash can, what does that say about her approach to her job? If she ignores it, what does *that* say? What about if she says, "Could you wait a minute for me, please? I need to call maintenance?"

While it oversimplifies matters to conclude anything concrete from her response, it does provide a clue. If she stops to pick up the pen, you might consider that she cares about the organization beyond her role in it; that she is a "detail" person; and that no task is too small for her to address when the need arises. If she ignores it, does that mean she does not care about much outside of her immediate interest and position? Could be. If she calls maintenance? Over a pen on the floor? You might be tempted to conclude she is just a bit officious—likes to throw her weight around.

Pick a scenario: She calls maintenance. How does that behavior square with your values and the kind of place you want to work? You are thinking, "*Really? She calls maintenance over a pen? Why doesn't she just pick it up and throw it away?*" Perhaps this organization has more structure, more hierarchy, and more defined limits on responsibilities than the dynamic, team-structured environment you were seeking.

What if she picked up the pen and you are thinking to yourself, "Why on earth would a VP ever stoop to do that? I am not doing that when I get to the executive level; that is why there are janitors." You might think twice before committing to this particular hospital, as it may say about you that you do not want to entertain this level of commitment to an organization; that you are more interested in status symbol reward than this organization provides. You may want a more hierarchical organization that limits individual responsibilities toward things not outside their direct purview.

No, you really cannot draw a hard-and-fast conclusion about the organization based on this behavior alone. But it provides a snapshot to include in examining other behaviors that, taken together, help describe an organization's culture. Understanding that culture and sensing whether you would thrive in it—or not—is what "good fit" is pretty much about.

THE OFFER AND ACCEPTANCE

You felt good about the two places you interviewed: BestintheCountry Health System (BCHS) and Outstanding Hospital. Then you received an offer from Outstanding Hospital. You talk with them about salary, health insurance, the 401(k), and relocation expenses, as we discussed in Chapter 8.

"I'M IN, MOM AND DAD! I'M GONNA START PAYIN' TAXES!"

You *accepted* the job. You are going to join Outstanding Hospital, a major teaching hospital that is planning and executing some innovative integration ideas. You call mom and dad with the good news. Clearly, *they* are relieved as you are no longer on their pay plan.

As a planning analyst at Outstanding, you will be in the thick of things. You were not certain about being in the western United States, but this is a great place with a great reputation and you liked the people. It is a good job, it will permit you to grow, the boss seems like a winner, and the pay is good. The people at BCHS, in the state next door to your home state where you also interviewed were just too late.

But before you called BCHS to tell them you just accepted an offer from Outstanding Hospital, they called you. "We were remarkably impressed with your talents; you interviewed extraordinarily well. We want to offer you the job." It is pretty much the same job as Outstanding Hospital's job. The pay is similar when you adjust for regional cost-of-living differences. But this is *BestintheCountry Health System*! There is no better place in the United States for care. BCHS is a leader in nearly every category of care and are on the cutting edge in a number of research activities. They not only *give* good care but they *define* it. Working there would look *great* on the résumé. And . . . and . . . it is only a short plane ride home.

What to do? Candidly, *you* should have never let it get this far. This is an ethical dilemma that has what most people believe is a right answer. When you accepted the position at Outstanding Hospital, you were telling them that you wanted to be a part of their organization. They indicated to you that they wanted you to be a part of the life of that organization and you agreed it was for you.

The second call you should have made—perhaps the third—after you accepted the job at Outstanding Hospital should have been to BCHS. (The first two calls are understandably to people you know who care about you and you care about them.) In that conversation with BCHS, you simply say, "I am honored to have been considered by BCHS and certainly did enjoy everyone I met there; however, I have accepted another offer." Short, sweet, to the point, and professional. They will appreciate the call. Will they be disappointed they missed out on hiring you? Perhaps. But there is little you can do about that. You needed to make a decision and you made the best decision you could have made at that time.

This simply cannot be overstated. Once you have accepted an offer of employment, you are ethically bound to see it through regardless of a subsequent job offer or opportunity to interview for something better. Not only is this (or at least should be) a matter of self-respect and respect for both your new employer and the one that came too late, but there is also a very practical reason for this. The business side of health care is a pretty small world. If you renege on your acceptance of employment at Outstanding Hospital, you will have burned the bridge, and in the process, you will have made several enemies. The hiring manager and a number of people involved in the process will remember your name—and not in a good way.

Let us play that thought out. Say the temptation is too much. You take the BCHS opportunity; call Outstanding Hospital and say "I am sorry, I have the chance to go to BCHS and I am going to take it." And so you go. After three to five years at BSHS, you decide you are ready to be a director of marketing. You apply to Greatcare Health System (GHS) in your home state only to discover that the VP for Strategy there is the former director of planning at Outstanding Hospital. He is the hiring manager you ended up cheating on about accepting the job he offered you. Uh oh. What do *you* think your chances are?

The example is a bit extreme to make a point. But it is a valid point nonetheless: by reneging on agreeing to take the job at Outstanding Hospital, you have, in effect, cheated. Your reputation will be damaged. It may never come to pass that you apply for a job where the people you cheated on would be doing the hiring, but they may know someone from Outstanding Hospital. People talk; people go to conferences to network; and people tell stories to one another about the good, the bad, and the ugly associated with their work. (That is partly why conferences exist!) You, and your name, will become one of those stories.

Once you commit, mean it. It is not a lifelong commitment, but it is a commitment to join the organization and do the very best job you can until such time as you have done all you can do there and feel the need to move on in order to face a greater challenge.

WHEW! I GRADUATED; GOT A GOOD JOB; AND KNOW EVERYTHING I NEED TO KNOW

Just because you received a sheepskin with some calligraphy and lettering in Latin does *not* mean you know everything you need to know. Hopefully, your education provided you some conceptual foundations and the ability to think critically in the milieu of health care management and policy. *That* was objective.

A professional is one whose work is derived from an intellectual achievement of both skills and knowledge, who applies that talent in service to others and for which the measurement of success is not necessarily monetary (Brandeis, 2010). *Part* of the intellectual achievement is complete—your degree. But your intellectual growth is by no means over.

As surely as night becomes day, change in how health care services are delivered will change over time. With those changes, people charged with managing the resources will need to grow in order to *lead* that change. It was not all that long ago, for example, that the predominant model in primary care delivery was the solo practitioner. He—and it was 99+% of the time a *he*—was the doctor; the wife was the office manager. Over time, for better or worse, the nature of practicing medicine became more complicated. Not only did the science change rapidly, but so did regulations, liability exposure, insurance payment systems, and greater encroachment into primary care by hospitals. Increasingly, it has become less possible for the solo practitioner working in the office with his wife to survive economically. Practices merged. Then merged again. Primary care doctors joined with specialists and vice versa. Hospital aggressively acquired both primary care and specialist practices in order to assure a flow of patients. Now the predominant model is hospital employment (Anthony R. Kovner & James R. Knickman, 2011). Practices are managed by professional managers.

Now the next phase of this development is gaining momentum—clinical integration. The advent of electronic records facilitates the movement of patient information from primary care doctor to specialist to the hospital, to the home health agency. Someone—managers—will need to understand this process inside and out in order to appropriately track costs and allocate resources.

If you expect to be successful in meeting the challenges of the future, you will need to know how to apply new information to the concepts you learned in school; you will need to take that critical thinking skill and apply it to a new set of circumstances to solve problems that did not exist 10 years ago. You will not be able to function in this world knowing only what you know today.

Continued active reading about the profession and its developments; going to conferences to attend sessions on what others are doing; leading conferences to share what you are doing and get feedback—these are all acts of lifelong learning. This is an integral part of professionalism—the ability and will to keep growing, developing, and learning.

ETHICAL CONSIDERATIONS OF SAYING "YES"

While it is beyond the purview of this book to articulate the entire range of ethical issues in the realm of health care administration, it is appropriate to highlight a few concepts that young professionals should bear in mind.

First, recognize that there are ethics, professional ethics, and laws. Ethics is the study of mores, customs, and behavior of a culture (Darr, 2005). Said another way, it is the study of how humans are in relationship with themselves and others (Baird, 2011). Of course, the study of ethics has been going on since the beginning of mankind, but it suffices to say here that there is the general concept of *ethics*, supplemented by a host of *professional* ethics—ethics for doctors, lawyers, and health services managers.

For us, as health care managers, we are concerned with issues that can be classified—though not in a particularly tidy way—as administrative and biomedical (Darr, 2005). In this vein, we are likewise concerned primarily with the autonomy of the patient and the relationship our organization has with the community at large. Clearly, we owe a duty to the patient. But do we owe a duty to the community and, if so, what is it? How do we understand what that obligation is?

As to the patient, what does it mean to assure the patient autonomy? For certain, that concept includes an informed consent, but does it include the right to die? If it does, then does it also imply an obligation on the part of health care providers to assist in bringing about that patient's death?

These are the kinds of questions we will not answer here. The point in surfacing them in this text is to make you better aware that each of us functions in a larger setting. How we relate to that setting—the community—is governed by principles ranging from those derivative of ancient philosophy to the Codes of Ethics promulgated by professional organizations. (You can find the ACHE Code of Ethics on the web by going to https://www.ache.org and searching for the Code of Ethics. Likewise, you can find the MGMA Code of Ethics by going to http://www.mgma.com and searching for Code of Ethics.)

Law is an embodiment of community norms. There are two ways to establish those norms. One is through the legislative process. When the legislature in a state establishes standards by which to license hospitals, it is codifying norms that the community expects to see in hospitals. The other way of embodying community norms is through the *common law*. This is a concept dating back to the seventeenth century in England. If there was a dispute in which one man injured another, the judge would look to the community to determine the normal circumstances that might occasion such an incident. Simply put, the judge looked to assess the community behavior and in so doing would find the law. Going forward then, this would be the standard for that community.

This might vary from state to state, community to community. In the realm of medical malpractice, for example, the community's expectation—the "standard of care" may be a bit stricter where there is access to an abundance of medical specialties and technology. You might find, for example, that in urban areas it is an expectation that a patient will be referred to a cardiologist for a routine 12-lead EKG. In rural areas, however, the standard might be that it is appropriate for a Family Practitioner to administer—and read—the 12-lead EKG simply because there are an insufficient number of cardiologists to adequately serve the community with that service.

In this way, our ethics are both incorporated into and bound by law. Is it possible to behave ethically and illegally at the same time? Is it possible to operate legally in a way that is unethical? Yes to both questions. The most desired state, of course, is to always engage in ethical behavior that is indisputably legal.

Observations from the Professionals

Giving Back to the Profession

Gayle L. Capozzalo, *FACHE is the Executive Vice President, COO and Chief Strategy Officer of the Yale-New Haven Health System. YNHHS is a 2,000 bed, three-hospital system serving southern Connecticut and is the clinical home for the Yale University School of Medicine. Ms. Capozzalo was the Chairperson of the American College of Healthcare Executives in 2012–2013.*

There is something incredibly special about health care that draws uniquely focused, determined, and passionate people to the field. In so many ways working in health care administration is an avocation driven by exceptional commitment and an underlying sense of purpose. It is a mission-driven profession that relies upon a solid foundation of integrity and lifelong learning. As the profession evolves, and we gain understanding of the importance of those we serve, the profession demands exceptional leadership and the recognition of the broad criticality of diversity.

As a result, giving back to the profession—and all that it offers us—is at the core of what we do.

As a young careerist, health care can provide wonderful mentors. Seek out those who have gained the strength of experience and ask for their guidance. Instead of shying away from the chaos that too often defines our environment, embrace it. Take on assignments that challenge you because in the uncertainty you can find direction. You will build confidence and understanding and develop a platform for future success.

As your career in health care progresses and you move into the senior ranks of the profession, there will be opportunities to assist those who follow in your steps. It is at the core of those who live the values of our profession to help others learn from their experience. All of us can recall people who have shaped our careers, provided timely advice and highlighted key elements of the problems we face. They provide a touchstone for the rest of our careers. They also can serve as exceptional examples of living the values of our work.

As a mentor, you can enhance your own coaching and leadership and management skills and bridge the gap between generations. Although the definition of a mentor often implies that the mentor is older than the protégé and always more experienced, it is important to point out that becoming a mentor may have more to do with having advanced experience and knowledge and wanting to share that with someone else rather than simply being older or at a higher level within an organization. Being more experienced can mean anything from offering advanced technical knowledge to listening skills. The concept can offer opportunities early in your career to not only be a protégé but to become a mentor.

It is all too easy to feel displaced by the growing complexity of health care. That is where the value of mentorship becomes most apparent. The nuance of the profession can feel overwhelming to even the more senior leaders among us. For those who must deal with the broadening gusts of change on a constant basis, a reliance on a personal and solidified code of ethics steadies us and provides us with the fortitude to make difficult decisions in the face of uncertainty. Integrity is a fundamental value of our profession.

Likewise, we must continue to grow and evolve to meet the rapidly shifting imperatives of the health care industry. Lifelong learning can be achieved in a variety of ways, but I have found enormous value through organizations such as the American College of Healthcare Executives (ACHE), which provides an important pathway toward improvement. ACHE is an international professional society for health care executives who lead hospitals, health care systems, and other health care organizations. It is the credentialing organization for the profession, offering the Fellowship (FACHE) credential signifying broad certification in health care management. It is never too early to engage with your colleagues to trade best practice, learn from examples, and broaden your horizon so it is important to explore organizations like ACHE early in your career. ACHE can provide opportunities for career development, career advancement, and continuing education through its publications, courses, research, and networks.

Lifelong learning can encourage you to look for opportunities, as your career develops, to teach in accredited health care management programs and provide opportunities for early careerists to network and learn about your organizations.

Much is made of leadership. Leadership is a learned attitude and skill. It is not dependent upon one's role in an organization or span of control. It is about inspiring, creating vision, listening, challenging, and facilitating. The health care industry is constantly changing and will continue to do so during your career. Ensuring that you continuously avail yourself of educational offerings in leadership, the health care industry, and organizational development is necessary to advance your career.

Giving back to your profession also includes becoming involved in the community in which you work and live. That involvement can evolve over time from volunteering at your children's school early in your career to becoming a leader in local and community government and not-for-profit organizations, church, etc. As a health care professional, community service should be an expectation. Representing your organization you can have a real and lasting impact on the people in your community.

Finally, embracing diversity from a personal and organizational perspective is both an ethical and a business imperative. Diversity in the health care profession serves as a catalyst for improved decision making, increased productivity, and better quality health care. Fostering an inclusive environment requires leadership that recognizes the contributions and supports the advancement of all, regardless of race, ethnicity, national origin, gender, religion, age, marital status, sexual orientation, gender identity or disability, because an inclusive environment can enhance the quality of health care, improve hospital/community relations, and positively affect the health status of society. Acting on the value of diversity requires asking difficult questions and challenging your individual and colleagues' assumptions. While mentoring, as mentioned earlier, is necessary for fostering leaders, the need for a mentoring program is especially acute for individuals of color and women.

Ensuring that you live on the professional values of integrity, lifelong learning, leadership, and diversity will provide you numerous opportunities to give back to the profession during your entire career.

EXERCISES

9-1 Find a fellow student colleague. Imagine an episode where the conduct of an administrator might be legal but unethical. How did they get to that situation? What could be done to avoid it?

9-2 Get with a partner. Imagine an episode where the conduct of an administrator might be ethical but illegal. How did they get to that situation? What could be done to avoid it?

9-3 Name a method of delivering care that is different today than it was 5 or 10 years ago. What is the procedure or drug? Why did this come into being? Now take that procedure or drug and consider it 10 years from now. Will it be the same? How might it be different?

9-4 You have just been offered a position with a major health organization—HSA "A." You ask them for a week to consider it to which they agree. In the meantime, you are in touch with another, bigger and better, health care organization, HSA "B" where you had also interviewed. The vice president making the decision at "B" is out of the office and not expected to return for three more days. You call "A" and ask for more time. They say "no" they really need to know by the end of the week. It becomes clear that you will not hear soon enough from "B." What do you do?

BIBLIOGRAPHY

Anthony R. Kovner & James R. Knickman, E. (2011). *Health Care Delivery in the United States (10th ed.)*. New York City: Springer Publishing.

Baird, C. (2011). *Everyday Ethics: Making Wise Choices in a Complex World*. Denver: Ethics Game Press.

Brandeis, L. D. (2010). 1912 Brown University Graduation Address. as quoted in *Good Business: Exercising Effective and Ethical Leadership at p. 10*. New York: Routledge.

Darr, K. (2005). *Ethics in Health Services Management (4th ed.)*. Baltimore, MD: Health Professions Press.

Chapter 10

Once You Are There (Internship, Residency or Job): Make It Count!

Wow! Your first job in your chosen profession! Congratulations. This is a terrific milestone. It is the culmination of years of hard work and diligent preparation.

(This chapter has been written as if the reader is in their first job or an administrative residency. Regardless of that, however, the principles and concepts here also apply to the student doing a summer internship or working at a part-time job while going to school. The fundamental message is "do everything you can to look, sound, and behave as if you are a professional," because—very simply—you are. The only question is where you are on the continuum in terms of professional development. You are a young professional as a new careerist; you are a developing professional as a student. In either case, the information in this chapter has currency for you.)

Now, however, is not the time to rest on your laurels. "What?!" you scream. "I need a break." Perhaps you can catch a few weeks between graduation and the beginning of work, but from now on you are probably looking at 48 to 52 weeks a year of work. Welcome to the real world. As many people may remind you, "Now you are a tax-paying citizen like the rest of us."

At the end of this chapter, students will understand business etiquette regarding management of time and consideration of others' time; will appreciate the importance of professional appearance; and will further understand the need to write and speak correctly. In addition, students will learn about the need to find a good mentor and develop a positive relationship with that person who can help them grow professionally. Finally, students will understand why it is important to continually seek challenging projects that will help them develop better and more varied skills, and that also increase their profile within the organization, and how that level of engagement can help lead to promotions.

BUILD A RELATIONSHIP WITH YOUR BOSS

This, of course, is the single most important thing you need to do. The process likely began during the interview process. This is a critically important person in your life at this juncture and the relationship with him or her requires careful attention and a thoughtful approach.

Know your boss' goals and align yours with them. Your number one job is to help him or her accomplish their goals. If they look good, you look good. Learn to anticipate their needs based on what they are trying to accomplish. If the priorities appear to be changing, ask. Sometimes the priorities can change rapidly and it is perfectly OK to ask about it so you can continue to be of help in a positive way. The bottom line here is simple: The more stuff you can keep off your boss' desk, the better for you both (assuming you do not cause a disaster in the process).

Get to know your boss' style. Some will want to micro-manage your work. Some will give you an excess of autonomy. In the case of the micro-manager, everything you do will be scrutinized to the *nth* degree. Do not take this personally. The boss who maximizes autonomy may well give you too much room. Do not take this personally, either. It does not mean your work is perfect. These are extreme cases, and there are still a few of both of these types out there, so be prepared. Most supervisors have figured out that an employee needs a certain degree of independence or empowerment to succeed in their role. Likewise, most also have learned that where there is no structure, there is no measureable progress.

Understand your boss' style. Is he amiable—interested in others? Is he analytical—loves to hunker over spreadsheets? Is he or she an extrovert or an introvert? None of these characteristics is, of course, mutually exclusive of the others. But there are traits that are more dominate, more noticeable than others. How will your style mesh with his? You may need to alter your approach to things in order to be more simpatico with your boss' style.

Keep these several things in mind:

- If you have 10 projects, your boss has 100.
- Sometimes when you ask for direction, you might not get as much as you think you need—the boss may want you to struggle a bit so you can learn.
- If you are having a meeting with the boss, prepare *thoroughly.*
- Respond to voice mails and e-mails from the boss ASAP—without exception.
- Do not be afraid to fail. That comes with the territory. The important thing is to learn from the mistake and not repeat it.
- Request a due date on all assignments.

- Do not miss the due date. If there will be a problem getting the project completed on time, inform the boss sooner rather than later and adjust the due date.
- Follow up. If you deliver, you will get more and better assignments.
- Do not build the watch; tell him the time. In other words, get to the point—always.
- Do not complain about a lack of resources. Are you being resourceful enough?
- If you did a lot of research for a memo or report, use an appendix. The boss does not need to wade through all that data in the middle of the text.

In summary, remember this one important fact: Your boss wants you to be successful. If he or she seems to be erecting barriers to what you think you need to be successful, the chances are they are challenging you to do better. They believe you can do better. The reason they want you to succeed is because it is also a reflection on them. Likewise, your success is, in part, tied to your boss' so do everything you can to learn his or her style and adapt to it.

BUY AN ALARM CLOCK; GET A DAILY ORGANIZER; BE PRESENT

Be on time by being at least five minutes early. If you have a meeting scheduled for 10 AM with the Administrative Director of Clinical Imaging, then do not show up at 10:05, saying "I forgot about the meeting." This will not help your career. By itself, will it sink you? Of course not. But it becomes a chink in the armor you do not need. Especially if this becomes a habit. Show up at 9:55 or 9:50.

One of the first things for you to understand is what time "the culture" of the organization requires you to be there. This may vary a bit by department, so pay close attention. Generally, the workday starts between 8 and 9 AM. In health care, especially hospitals, the work frequently starts closer to 7 or 8 AM than 9. There are several reasons for this: Doctors make their rounds early and if you expect to see one of them regarding a committee on which you are serving together, then early is the time to catch them. Otherwise, they will be in clinic all day with patients and will have no time for administrative functions. Breakfast meetings with doctors are common in the hospital setting. The other reason things begin early in the morning is that nurses usually have shift change around 7 or 7:30. While this will seldom involve you directly, that activity seems to send a charge of energy through the organization and it just feels right to be there.

Once you determine when you need to show up for work, map how long it will take you to get there from your home. Do you need to take a train? A bus? How long is the drive? The other excuse you do not want to use is "I got stuck in traffic." Absent a major pile-up on a thoroughfare you absolutely must take to get to work, all this says is that "I did not plan my time appropriately." This is where you need to own the consequences of your actions. Be sure to leave plenty of time to get to work on time. Indeed, get there early so you can get settled in before getting on with the day's work.

If you do not already have an appointment calendar, get one or start using the calendar on your smartphone. There is seldom a good excuse for forgetting about a meeting and either missing it or being late for it. Organizations of all sizes have plenty of meetings; some are formal, some informal. This depends on the organization. You will spend a good amount of time in meetings, so have a good system to keep track. You can keep a calendar on your laptop that syncs with your smartphone; you can keep a hand written one that you carry with you. You can get a desk calendar that lets you make notes and add a to-do list and so forth. It does not matter which one you prefer. Just be sure to have a calendar and use it for everything. Most organizations now have a calendar on their e-mail systems that you can sync to your smartphone, so when you agree in the hallway to meet with someone on the second Tuesday of next month at 10 AM, you can record it instantly in your smartphone for automatic updating of your laptop calendar. Likewise, in that same conversation if you need to refer back to a meeting that took place last

week, you can do that as well. Smartphones are terrific tools. They are much more than micro-screens for gamers or another version of MP3. Use yours to keep track of your time so you will know where you belong and when.

The advice about showing up early for the interview has some application here. It is best to show up a few minutes early for a meeting. You do not need to arrive 30 minutes before so you can shine the boss' shoes, but getting there five minutes early is always a good idea. It prevents you from being late; and you may get some additional face time with the person calling the meeting.

Be present refers to your mental approach to the meeting. Focus on the agenda items. Soak up all the information you can; learn from what is being said. If you have an idea or good thought, understand the culture of the organization to determine if you should share it. But if it is permissible, then by all means, do speak up. Engage. Take good notes. Be a part—an active part—of the process.

APPEARANCE COUNTS

There is an old saying that probably is true: "The job candidate will never look any better than he does when he interviews." If you think on some level that it is OK to go casual, or even business casual, now that you have the job, think again. When you went to the interview, you should have taken note about the culture, including among other things, the way people dress for work. Hospitals are often culturally conservative organizations, and professional dress is nearly always a must. Employees at consulting firms, on the other hand, frequently are dressed in business casual when they are in the office and only dress in full professional uniform when they have client meetings or other professional meetings outside of the office. Nonclinical professionals working in physician offices are often in attire that is mixed between business casual and professional, while professionals in long-term care generally dress either in business casual or full business professional. So understand the culture of the organization and dress accordingly.

Dress the way the next level of management above you dresses. You do not want to be in an entry-level position for longer than necessary, right? One way to send the signal that you are ready to be elevated to better, higher-level challenges is to *look* like you are ready. Granted, it is more about skills, knowledge, and ability when organizations think about moving people ahead. You will not get promoted on your good looks. But looking the part never got anyone held back, whereas failure to look the part most certainly will be a detriment to the knows-it-all-but-looks-like-a-slob geek. If you want to be an administrative director, then dress like an administrative director; when you get to that level and you want to be a vice president, then dress like a vice president.

COMMUNICATE: DO IT WELL AND DO IT WITH STYLE

The failure to communicate clearly leads to more mistakes, mishaps, and errors, than you can count. Communication requires care and attention to detail. There are, of course, both written and oral communications. The memo, the e-mail, and the report are all basic tools of the trade for transmitting information. Likewise, the phone call, the meeting, and the one-on-one meeting all are critically important for management to move the organization in its chosen direction to successfully perform its mission.

The Spoken Word: Listen Carefully

The first thing anyone must do in sharing information orally is . . . *listen*. Nature gave you two ears and one mouth and it works best if you use them in roughly that proportion. Listening is more than hearing. It is the process of learning from what is being spoken by another. In the context of work, you should be an active listener. Ask questions if you are uncertain about what is being said. Ask questions if you want to know more about a particular point—be curious. When you listen actively, you are demonstrating to the speaker that you are engaged in what she is saying. Likewise, when you ask questions, it displays your interest in growing professionally, as you are implicitly saying "I would like to know more." Hear and consider the information or the ideas. The fact that you are intently listening, as evidenced by your demeanor as well as the questions you ask, will encourage the speaker to be comfortable and more candid with you. So ask questions. Of course, this does not mean to behave like your two-year old nephew: "Why is the sky blue?," "Why is dirt brown?," "Why, why why . . ." "Why are you gritting your teeth and looking at me like that, Ms. Jones?" The point being, do not ask questions just for the sake of asking questions in the belief that you can never go wrong in doing this. Ask questions if you are genuinely uncertain about what is being said, or if you are truly curious about how or why something is a particular way.

The Spoken Word: Do Not Just Spit It Out

Before you say a thing—*think*. If you are presenting information, do it from the ground up. That is to say, give the most basic information first, and then build up to the details. No need to break the human record for most words in a minute, either. Speak slowly enough that you can properly enunciate the words, (but not so slowly that you sound like the Slo-Mo replay on a sports' show highlight reel). Make sure the listener is getting a basic understanding of what it is that you are trying to convey.

Second, like the interview and like any presentation you have ever done, use the tone of your voice and body language to underscore certain points. Some of the things you are saying are more important than others. Let the listener know that by modulating the tone of your voice. If you just speak in a monotone (a) everyone in the room will know you do not care about the subject and (b) will be either nodding off or daydreaming about being—anywhere—else. Make the subject more interesting and emphasize certain points by varying the tone of your voice and moving your hands. No need to flail about like a conductor at the symphony, but just use some movement of your hands to provide emphasis.

This is one of the hardest things for some people: Look the person to whom you are speaking in the eye. Just like the interview, this is important to establish credibility—and to get the point across. It conveys your interest in the subject and the listener. You will be able to read the listener by looking them in the eye. Just like the interview, break eye contact on occasion. It is not a stare down contest.

Reaffirm that the listener is getting the drift of what you are saying by asking a question or two to elicit a response. Even a simple "Does that seem plausible?" or "Do you see my point?" goes a long way to demonstrate to the listener that you want to be sure they understand. They will appreciate the fact that you care about their level of understanding.

Finally, encourage others to share perspective and ideas. Whatever it is that you are talking about there is more than one way to see it. Your view of the topic was most certainly not handed down by Moses engraved in stone. Neither is anyone else's, so it is always good to generate additional ideas both on the merits of solving whatever the problem at hand is, as well as stylistically from the standpoint of being engaging and receptive from the listener's perspective.

The Written Word

This is a critically important skill, a good bit of which was addressed in Chapter 2. Chances are you will be writing memos, reports, and e-mails (which are more frequently substituting for memos) for the consumption of others. If you are merely reporting on an outcome of a project, or if you are advocating for one particular course of action over another, the structure and coherency of your writing will bear on one thing at the very least: your credibility.

First, determine the audience. Is this a single person? Should other people be included? Should those people also be primary addressees or merely copied on the missive? Include only those who *need* to be included; do not include everyone in second tier management.

Second, have a clean, clear heading. Check with someone else in the organization. See if there is a standard format in use. If not, develop your own memo template. You can add this as a macro to your computer so you do not have to redo it every time you write a memo.

Start with the conclusion, for example, "The purpose of this memo is to summarize the cost-benefit analysis of acquiring a new 3.0 Tesla MRI." This is brief and to the point.

Then discuss the issue. In our example, you would want to calculate the potential revenue that could be generated by this high-powered device. Then develop the cost of acquisition. One general word of advice on these kinds of questions: Always try to estimate the minimal amount of revenue and the maximum possible cost. This is *not* to say you should be misleading! You should not! But there is usually a range of highs and lows in making these kinds of estimates. It is appropriate to point that out that you have adopted a conservative posture by projecting the maximum cost and the minimum revenue. Look at it this way: If the device can be profitable under *these* circumstances, it will do very well financially if you are too aggressive in estimating costs or too timid in projecting revenue.

Following the discussion, you should have a brief summary. "Based on this analysis, the 3.0 Testla MRI would greatly expand our ability to produce images of prostate and breast cancers, thereby improving both the quality of care we provide and the number of patients we could serve."

And if the circumstances call for it, then the last paragraph should be a concluding recommendation.

One last word about memos (more on e-mails below): Keep it as brief as possible. You will earn high marks from those who need to read them if you can stay within a one-page limit. Remember the audience is a very busy person or group of busy people. If they can glean what they need to know from a single page memo, they will appreciate the fact that you saved them time from having to read more.

You can use this same basic structure for reports and e-mails as well. But keep in mind, if you do not write well, then all the structure in the world will not help make a memo better.

PROJECTS AND MENTORS

The late Zig Ziglar, a former pots and pan salesman turned motivational speaker, had a tremendous gift for inspiring people to achieve more. One of the many quotes people have taken from his speeches is this: "If you want more, do more."(Ziglar, 1977). It has application here because either you are seeking an entry-level position to begin your professional career or you are looking to move beyond your first job. Presumably, you do not want to stay in that "entry level" mode any longer than you have to, so, for you to move up in the organization, you need to do more.

The practical implication of this is the simple advice to seek out more and better projects on which to work and do the very best you can on the projects to which you are assigned. You may start out coordinating a special event for the organization to participate in a large charity, for example. Do not treat this lightly! Your challenge is to exceed the prior level of participation however it may be measured—by dollar contributions or number of participants. Take the challenge *con brio* as they say in music: with zest. Do not feel like you are the last person on the totem pole assigned to a challenge no one else wanted. Rather, view this as (1) an opportunity to meet a large number of people within the organization and (2) a leadership opportunity to improve the organization's posture in the community. A former student received a post-graduate fellowship at a very prominent, large health care organization on the East Coast. He was assigned responsibility for the organization's participation in United Way. He was miffed and basically told his supervisors, "I don't want to do this; that isn't why I got my MHA." He was gone within six months, well ahead of the scheduled end date for his fellowship.

It is likely true, however, since you are reading this book, that you may not have much interest in organizing your employer's charity special events the rest of your career. For that reason, not only do you want

to demonstrate that you can do a terrific job on the task you have been assigned, but you want to seek out more interesting and challenging projects as well. Do not hesitate to go to your supervisor and ask for *additional* projects. If you have a project that is near the end point, give your leadership a heads-up that you will need a replacement project in the near future.

How do you determine if a project is a good project? First, it needs to generally fit your skill set. If you have been asked to assess the clinical and business ramifications of building a new multi-specialty clinic on the other side of town, consider saying "no." This project is too big; requires too many different skill sets and, therefore, is not a good project. It is one at which you most certainly would fail, unless you are providing staff support for a larger committee or task force of more senior people. A good project would be if you were asked to study and report on how the distribution of physicians holding clinic would change if that multi-specialty clinic gets built. What makes this a good project is that it utilizes your skill set; you can do the spreadsheets and engage your interpersonal skills as you communicate with others. Connecting with others is the other element that makes this a good project: you cannot do it alone. You will need some advice from the practice administrator; you will need some advice from the financial division; you most certainly will need advice from physicians. In other words, this is a project that will force you into places outside of your comfort zone, but not so far out of it that you are sure to fail. This project will require you to match up quantitative analysis with the human dimension, for example. Part of this notion of professional growth is to get projects like this and then get to the right people to ask questions. (That's another reason that charity event is not a bad beginning point; you will get acquainted with a variety of people from across the organization.) If you go to your boss and ask for a project and she responds with something that you *think* you can do, but are not certain; when you think you want to say "I don't know, but I can give it a try." *that* is a good project. The third aspect of what makes a good project is the profile it provides for you. Are you going to have the opportunity to report on your findings to a team of other, higher level administrators? That is a good thing. A report that will be used as a source in a larger document being prepared by your boss, from a profile perspective, is not a great project. It is, however, one of those projects discussed above, do it very well so your boss will be confident in giving you higher profile responsibilities.

Perhaps one of the most important things you can do as an entry level employee in any organization is to find a mentor within the organization. This should be a person who has several—if not many—years of experience in the profession and at the organization where you are working. It need not be your direct supervisor. It does not need to be anyone in the chain of command of your position. Indeed, it is probably better if the person is outside that chain of command.

You are looking for a person who can offer an objective assessment of any situation that you present to them. You are looking for someone who can explain a different perspective if you have encountered something especially vexatious. This should be someone you can trust; someone to whom you can take problems to ask for advice. This is not to say that you need your mother in this role. You do not need someone to provide you a crying towel every time you hit a bump in the road. You need someone to explain why the bump is there and what you need to do to get past it as smoothly as possible. The mentor's gender does not matter; however, even in the twenty-first century, women's issues in the workplace may be, and often are, different from some of the issues confronted by men, so a female mentor may have special importance to the young woman professional.

MEETING ETIQUETTE: HOW TO AVOID UNWANTED ATTENTION

This is important material for some of you as you may not have experienced many meetings in professional settings. Perhaps your most common exposure to the analog of professional meetings

is going to class. One of the things many of you do, that you believe is beyond faculty's ability to notice, is socialize through your Facebook page while sitting in the back row. (Please observe that "you believe is beyond faculty's ability to notice" carefully.)

You *were* noticed by your faculty (if you were one of these people), and you most certainly will be noticed by your professional colleagues if you pull this kind of sophomoric stunt on the job. Simply put, *during meetings do not:*

- Be online with Facebook, LinkedIn, Twitter, or any other social media sites unless it is necessary to getting an answer to a question that arose during the meeting.
- Call someone on your phone; answer the phone. Do neither of these. Put the phone on Airplane mode or shut it off.
- Initiate or answer e-mail. The same applies to texts and tweets.
- Twiddle your thumbs, crack your knuckles, or engage in any of those nervous tic-like behaviors.
- Roll your eyes, frown, or make other facial expressions expressing boredom or negative judgment.

On the other hand, *during meetings you should:*

- Pay close attention: again, this can be a learning opportunity.
- Like the interview; lean in a bit to show interest.
- Ask questions of things you do not understand.
- Offer constructive ideas and comment when appropriate.

THE USE (AND MISUSE) OF E-MAIL: A CONSUMER'S GUIDE TO ETIQUETTE

E-mail seems like the opening line from *A Tale of Two Cities* sometimes: "It was the best of times. It was the worst of times" (Dickens, 1859). It is a terrific tool that has helped flatten the hierarchy of organizations everywhere. It facilitates the transmission of information around the globe nearly instantaneously. It makes it possible to stay in closer touch with more people, across a greater geographic expanse than anything known to man before it arrived. Likewise, it is driving managers everywhere nuts. E-mail has led to information overload; shirking of job responsibilities; and eliminated other superior forms of communication such as face-to-face or telephone calls, replacing quality with convenience. It invites spuriousness and unneeded duplication. It has compounded the damage done by wasting time. It produces a false sense of the "need for speed." (You, of course, think e-mail is burdensome and too slow because you text at the speed of light and expect the same of everyone else.)

The fact is we do too much by e-mail. It is not uncommon for an executive or upper-level manager to have 200 e-mails a day. Assuming one minute to dispense with each, that would be 3 hours and 20 minutes out of that person's day to deal with this infernal mess. By the same token there is likely some good information among those 200 e-mails; and the executive's response will be far-reaching in its consequences. Of course, with 200 mails in her inbox the executive might well overlook or miss the consequences of the two or three most important among them.

There are a few rules that will stand you in good stead with your colleagues in the workplace.

1. *Respect Recipient's Time.* Take a few extra minutes if necessary to reduce your message to the most succinct possible. Again, particularly for you in an entry-level position, you will be writing to people who are as busy as someone trying to drink water from a fire hydrant. Keep it short.

2. *Do Not Write or Reply in Haste.* If you are responding to an e-mail from someone else, you need not do it within five minutes of the time you received it. Do be prompt, but take some time to be thoughtful in your response. Be accurate rather than too fast. Consider the consequences beyond yourself. Also, if initiating an e-mail because you are angry, do not send it. When he was angry, Abraham Lincoln wrote letters that he never sent (Goodwin, 2005). It is a good rule. Apply it to e-mail. If you send off an electronic version of the middle finger, you *will* regret it.

3. *Be Clear.* Use the subject line to describe "Not Urgent," "Time Sensitive," "Action required." Use one or two additional words to capture the subject. For example: "Action required: MRI Acquisition." In the body of the e-mail, use crisp sentences and keep the length to a bare minimum. If it takes more than a couple of paragraphs, consider sending a memo as an attachment. Keep the overall look clean by avoiding goofy fonts and artsy background and graphics.

4. *Be Specific with Questions.* Again, consider the audience. If you are writing to describe several options for a decision, do not end it with "Your thoughts?" or "Let me know how I can help." Those things are entirely too general. If you want to offer to help, outline several options: "Can I help by (a) calling the vendor; (b) scheduling a time for the vendor to visit; or (c) would you prefer I not be involved?" is an example of a far better approach.

5. *Do Not Copy Unneeded Recipients.* Not everyone in the Western world needs to see the wisdom you have inscribed in pixels on a screen. Just *copy* the people who actually are involved who *need* to see it. If you can, avoid "Reply to All." If you are being asked to join a meeting with 20 other people, only the originator needs to know you are out on Thursday, but available on Tuesday and Wednesday PM.

6. *Cut the Threads.* One of the largest pet peeves for managers and executives is to receive an e-mail that reads something like this: "Please see the conversation below. Thoughts?" followed by a thread of multiple e-mails. Really?! It is *your* job to scale all that information down to a manageable amount and then offer to help in a specific way. If you cannot do that, consider scheduling a phone conversation.

7. *Minimize Attachments.* Avoid using logos or signatures that appear as attachments. These things

use up memory on the server, slow down the performance of the recipient's computer, and add no value to the communication.

8. *Be Brief—Part Two.* If you can convey something in five or six words, put it in the subject line followed by EOM (end of message). That way the recipient does not need to take the time to open the message. Likewise, you can add NNTR (no need to reply) to the end of your messages if you do not need a response. An example: "Here is an additional item for tomorrow's agenda. NNTR."

9. *Avoid Responses That Have No Meaning.* "Thanks!"—everyone knows you are grateful. If you receive a bit of information (like "I'll be in tomorrow at 11. We can meet then.") you do not need to respond at all, including "Great!"

10. *Avoid Using for Confidential Matters.* Do not put anything in an e-mail that you would be uncomfortable reading in a newspaper. Do not use e-mail to discuss sensitive personnel matters. Do not use e-mail to discuss questions of legal liability or matters that would embarrass the organization (or you) if subsequently discovered by others. It is too easy to forward information into the hands of those who should not have it. It is too easy to find incriminating information in the event of litigation.

11. *Take a Break from Electronic Media.* It will be helpful for you if you try using the phone a bit more often. It would be healthy if you get away from electronic media on weekends, or at least for part of the weekends.

A Note About Telephone Etiquette

On a peripheral matter, take good care of your telephone etiquette as well. Do not eat, chew gum or yawn when you are on the phone. Update your recorded greeting from time to time. Keep the greeting simple, as well: name and a brief statement about when you will return the call. Avoid all the gimmicks like sound effects and celebrity voices (Stafford, 2012).

CONCLUSION

Professional demeanor is a critically important part of career planning and development. It is not as if one will get promoted simply because they look and sound the part. It does not work that way. The material in this chapter speaks to the notion of how to best present your skills, knowledge, and ability— the things that are assessed and considered by organizations when considering promotions. There is no substitute for competence! But competence can be more easily seen when presented in a way that makes it easy to see. A genius who writes a five-page memo to describe a process that could have been reduced to one or two pages may get credit for having a penchant for detail, but the person who can reduce complexity to its basics and act on them is demonstrating more: an ability to think critically and minimize demand on the upper echelon of leadership.

The ways in which you conduct yourself in meetings, on the phone, in presentations, and in e-mails are all a part of your appearance to others in the workplace. From this chapter you should have developed a sound set of ideas about how to handle the everyday situations in the workplace. While none of these things, standing alone, will kill, sidetrack, or advance your career, they do, when taken together, establish a persona that will very much be a part of determining where you can take your career.

Observations from the Professionals

The Most Important Things to Do When You Get There

Emily Hardeman *is an associate project director in the Office of the Senior Vice President and Chief of Clinical Operations at The University of Texas MD Anderson Cancer Center. Located in Houston, TX, MD Anderson is one of the world's most respected centers devoted exclusively to cancer patient care, research, education, and prevention.* U.S. News & World Report's *"Best Hospitals" survey ranked MD Anderson as the top hospital in the nation for cancer care in 2011. Ms. Hardeman completed her Administrative Fellowship at MD Anderson prior to entering into her current position.*

Starting off in a fellowship program or first job can be exciting, energizing, and downright daunting all at the same time. As an early careerist, I have found that you have to completely step outside of your comfort zone and be open to any and all opportunities you may come across. As cliché as this all may sound, being present is incredibly important; arrive early, stay late, and be around to participate whenever something comes your way. No matter how insignificant an event or meeting may seem, whether in or out of work, attending these events and networking with other professionals may help you gain knowledge and advance in your career.

Life was glamorous during our fellowship year. We were able to attend high-profile meetings, functions, office parties, etc., so we really did experience a move to the "dark side" during our first jobs post-fellowship. When you go from working on high-level institutional initiatives to departmental projects and research that may go unnoticed, you learn very quickly that you have to check your ego at the door and start at the bottom; we must all remember that we are not too big for anything. You will see people climb the ladder very quickly, with or without justification, and it is so easy to begin comparing yourself to others and where you would like to be, but your career is your own, so worry about yourself—be present, network, work hard, and avoid burning bridges.

Always be open and willing to take on new projects that will not only benefit your organization, but your own personal and professional development as well. It is hard to say "no" when everybody wants a fellow's labor, but be careful not to overextend yourself to the point where your work is not reflective of your potential. Additionally, do not avoid smaller projects that may appear menial, for these are the projects that you can make your own and build your reputation. I was fortunate to have a preceptor who helped develop a challenging, yet achievable workload, in order to allow time for *ad hoc* assignments and meetings from which I could benefit. Identifying and engaging with a mentor is crucial to one's continued success, as these are the individuals who will help to identify, and teach you how to manage, small projects that may evolve into high impact projects.

I always felt like I had been a team player, but I cannot stress the importance of encouraging positive group dynamics as you are starting off your career. Whether you are paired up with other fellows on projects, sharing an office with a coworker, or participating in a meeting, the impressions you make on others during the first few years may impact your relationships and recruitment opportunities for years to come. Do not get me wrong; a little competition is healthy, as you must make yourself stand out amongst potential hiring managers; however, collaborating amongst peers also stands out. Learn from your peers and use them as sounding boards. Working with a group of fellows, I can't tell you how many times I read an e-mail aloud or proofed a write-up to ensure the point was made in a clear and concise manner.

One of the hardest things for me about working with a group of fellows was not being able to control our schedule. I am typically about 10 minutes early to any meeting or event, but when you are expected as a group, you must wait for the group. My peers labeled my walk the "mom walk" because I was always trying to get us to rotations on time; in the end, that walk almost always helped to get us there on time! Regardless of whether you are meeting with the CEO or a group of students, always try to respect their time and provide your undivided attention while doing so. There is nothing worse than meeting with someone who e-mails and answers pages during the entire meeting. I get it—we work with physicians, who HAVE to answer certain pages—but the rest of us can probably get by for 10–15 minutes without stepping out of the room!

Speaking of respect, try your best to look the part. You are representing all fellows that came before you and all that will come after you. You are representing young graduates in the workplace. I am not saying spend a fortune on clothes or hours in front of the mirror, but if you are attending high-level meetings and participating in institutional projects and initiatives, look like and act like a professional.

EXERCISES

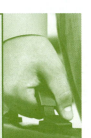

10-1 Get a partner and attend a meeting of some kind. It can be the Health Professions club or a student government meeting or some other kind of topic-related group or service organization. Take notes. Do not share your notes with your partner; do not discuss the meeting between yourselves. Write a one-page detailed summary of the meeting, as if you were writing to inform someone (your boss?) who did not attend. Share with your partner and critique each other's work. Did you capture the important details of the meeting? Does your partner think you captured the important parts?

10-2 Select an upcoming day, perhaps a Saturday or Sunday. Turn off your computer, tablet, smartphone, and any other electronic communications media. Leave them off for a 24-hour day. Make some notes at the end of the day about how that felt; share with a friend who has done the same thing.

BIBLIOGRAPHY

Dickens, C. (1859). *A Tale of Two Cities.* London: Chapman & Hall.

Goodwin, D. K. (2005). *Team of Rivals.* New York: Simon & Schuster.

Stafford, D. (2012, July 2). Better Business Phone Etiquette. *The (Charleston, SC) Post and Courier*, pp. D-11.

Ziglar, Z. (1977). *See You at the Top.* New Orleans: Pelican Publishing Co.

Chapter 11

What It Is Like to Be in the Profession

"I WONDER WHAT IT WOULD BE LIKE TO BE . . ."

Students may often wonder what it must be like to be a hospital executive, or a pharmaceutical sales representative, or to be in some other role in the health care industry. This chapter attempts to provide a partial answer to that question. Unlike the other chapters, there are no exercises for this chapter and there will be no conclusion. Here you will find a collection of essays from a variety of non-clinical health care professionals that describe some of what they do on a daily or routine basis. At the end of the chapter, you will have a better understanding of the professional lives of people from different segments of the health care industry.

A DAY IN THE LIFE OF AN EXECUTIVE DIRECTOR AT A CONTINUING CARE RETIREMENT COMMUNITY

Jacque Richardson is Executive Director, The Lakes at Litchfield (SC). Jacque has devoted her entire professional career to medical service industry, ranging from acute and post-acute care, home health, and long-term care. She is a strong proponent of continuing education and believes that "textbooks" provide a firm foundation. She also feels that the actual work environment is the real "teacher" where one can employ the knowledge that is written.

Learning something new almost every day is the best part of my professional career; if you have stopped learning it is time to move on. I know the importance of furthering your career with continuous learning and surrounding yourself with individuals who are also ready to take on any challenge. Every morning when I step through the front doors of our community, I know I will be presented with a new challenge and I am excited to take it head on.

The number one goal at the Lakes at Litchfield, owned and operated by Senior Living Communities, is to help Members live longer, healthier, and happier lives. Through award-winning wellness programs, dedication to preparing and serving fantastic food, the ability to provide services allowing people to stay independent in their own home and by abiding by the simple rule of treating others like we want to be treated, the Lakes at Litchfield is giving people the ability to live a higher quality of life.

I have never worked with any company that is willing to invest whatever it takes to razzle-dazzle our customers. At Litchfield, we have the best customer service and training that I have been a part of in my 30+ years of geriatric training.

As a Continuing Care Retirement Community (CCRC), The Lakes at Litchfield offers all levels of care from independent cottages and apartments to assisted living, including memory care and skilled nursing. People do not understand what we do. Physicians do not understand it and families certainly do not. There is an assumption that either we are a nursing home or everything falls under the umbrella of assisted living.

The Lakes at Litchfield is redefining senior housing. We are constantly planning on how we can improve current services and offer new services, while keeping ourselves competitive in the market. Members of all community neighborhoods, including independent living, assisted living, skilled nursing, and Alzheimer's care, are able to enjoy an all-inclusive, maintenance free lifestyle. Amenities include restaurant-style dining, housekeeping, residential and lawn maintenance, daily activities, exercise, and wellness programs and included utilities.

We have proven that people who come into these types of communities are living longer. We have members who have lived here since our doors opened 17 years ago. We have four centurions; two of them are still living in their independent apartments. The driving force behind every service at Litchfield is The Weller Life®. Senior Living Communities and The Lakes at Litchfield firmly believe that people at any age, at any condition, at any point in their life can get better and can actually improve their health, fitness level, and wellness level.

Wellness is not just a buzzword. We do not simply throw a piece of equipment in a room and say that we have got a wellness program. We have dedicated wellness professionals from Life Enrichment Leaders to our Wellness Director where stand-alone centers may only have one person who is their activity person.

The community was the recipient of the Assisted Living Federation of America (ALFA) Best of the Best awards in 2010 for the WAVES program. That important program helps those suffering from Alzheimer's disease and dementia by reducing agitation, increasing appetite, and improving sleep patterns. The community was again selected in 2011 for C.L.I.M.B., which aims to improve one's confidence, longevity, independence, mobility, and balance and yet a third time in 2012 for Purpose-Based Wellness Programs.

One thing I find in this business is that the people who work in it have a passion. It is not just work. Our entire team feels the same way. When I arrived in September 2009, I had to build a new team. You have to hire right, train, and retain. My hires have proven to be successful because we were awarded Senior Living Communities' Community Supernova award in 2011 and 2013. Surrounding yourself with good people is the ticket for your success in this business.

A big part of why we have been successful is our emphasis on employee retention. The community offers various programs catering to employees of all levels from the Track to Success for Certified Nursing Assistants and Frontline Leaders to Elevate, which provides student loans for continued education to Evolve, the Executive Director Training Program.

I am a firm believer in participative management. I believe in giving power away. Managing in a dictatorial, fear fashion is not a healthy thing. I give my team a lot of rope. While I may have to pull the rope in at times, I always try to use those instances as teachable moments.

I have an open door policy, which extends to more than simply having my office door open. I situate my desk so that I can see the entire business office area at the community and I am reachable by phone 24 hours a day. One thing the members will tell you is that I am very accessible and very responsive.

At all Senior Living Communities, the sales people are given the job title Lifestyle Advisor. I believe everyone at the community advises on the retirement lifestyle. When people come to us, particularly with adult children, there is a lot of guilt. They desperately want to care for their parent; however, distance or work prevents them from doing so. We have to put ourselves in their shoes and show empathy.

Education and Professional Background

My geriatric career started at Columbia College where I graduated with a double major in Social Work and Psychology. My undergraduate degree has helped me tremendously. It is a good foundation for being able to do what I am currently doing. After graduation, I worked as a Medical Social Worker for the Marion County Hospital System.

While at Marion, I worked a lot with the geriatrics through nursing home placements, plans for them to go home, home health referrals, hospice care, and medical equipment. I was fortunate enough to work hand in hand with the physicians. They trained me and trusted me to work outside my assigned job duties. While working in this full-time position, I obtained a Master's of Science in Health Services Administration from the Medical University of South Carolina.

After working as a Medical Social Worker for 13 years, I decided I was ready for the next challenge. For that reason, I reached out to my hospital CEO about other positions or added responsibilities and was presented with the challenge to recruit physicians for the hospital. Knowing how difficult it would be to bring anyone to Marion County, I was ready to take on this opportunity. In 24 months, I recruited numerous positions and helped these physicians open and run their local practices.

During my tenure with the hospital, the company bought a local nursing home that was deemed for closure by the Department of Health and Environmental Control (DHEC). The nursing home was in need of a complete overhaul. The hospital asked me to sit for the Nursing Home Administrators' exam. Upon passing, a young RN and I were able to get the nursing home out of trouble. We worked closely with the regulatory agencies, which proved to be very supportive and helpful during this process.

I later pursued a career in a start-up Home Health Agency. Through much hard work and dedicated staff, we accomplished a thriving business within the first quarter of opening.

After, I took a brief hiatus from the corporate world opting for freelance work and consulting for local long-term care facilities.

In 2002, I joined the world of retirement communities by serving as Executive Director for a CCRC out of Greenville, S.C. I worked there until 2009 when I was recruited by Senior Living Communities to work at their Brightwater community in Myrtle Beach to get the new Assisted Living and Skilled Nursing running, licensed, and hire a team. I worked with Brightwater for six months before being asked to become the Executive Director of The Lakes at Litchfield.

A DAY IN THE LIFE OF A BUSINESS OPERATIONS MANAGER AT A MID-SIZED COMMUNITY HOSPITAL

Bill Burmeister is currently the Business Operations Manager Middlesex Hospital in Middletown, CT, reporting directly to the Chief Nursing Officer in an oversight and advising role of all budgetary, operational, billing, and clinical support areas of inpatient nursing. Middlesex Hospital is a Magnet-designated, Top 100, acute care hospital with 275 licensed beds, 3 satellite emergency departments, and a large number of hospital-owned physician practices and outpatient facilities. Bill began with the organization as an Administrative Fellow prior to his current role immediately after graduating from Pennsylvania State University with his MHA in 2009.

At Middlesex Hospital, I am responsible for a $30 million operating budget and have implemented several new strategies to combat rising labor costs across the organization. Some of these initiatives include the formation of an internal nursing float pool, the implementation of a hospital-wide, web-based scheduling system, several process efficiency enhancements, including a central transportation dispatch model, and new strategies to manage productivity and budget variance levels on all units.

Other responsibilities of mine include advising all nurse managers on budgetary and billing issues, holding introductory finance and budgeting courses as well as process improvement seminars for nursing unit councils, and developing and presenting all labor and capital requests for most inpatient departments. Previous to the development of my role, these were all responsibilities shared amongst nursing department managers and directors, which created differing opinions and a decentralized approach to process redesign and budgeting.

At the time I was offered the position, the role was still fairly new for the organization, and without a clinical background I was certainly weary of the challenges ahead. Given the organization had consistently been a top clinical performer in the country among community hospital peer groups, receiving numerous awards and designations along the way, I knew that a stronger business presence without a clinical history would prove challenging at first. Whenever I presented expense-reduction opportunities or process efficiency improvements, the response from front line clinical staff and management was generally focused on patient care, quickly shifting away from my comfort zone of operations. Just to be clear, by no means do I believe this tendency is undesirable or needless, but it can certainly prove to be an unmanageable barrier if you do not listen and seek input from all stakeholders. With that said, I learned to develop a much stronger appreciation for all caregivers and their dedication to their patients. No nurse wants to hear about why we cannot offer his or her patient round the clock meals, more staff, better rooms, or certain supplies, and even more importantly, they do not want to hear it from someone with a primarily business background.

The challenge with all of my work is in balancing the clinical goals of the nursing department with the financial objectives of the organization. On the surface, they appear to be competing purposes, but if planned and communicated appropriately, the two can certainly complement each other. For example, staffing and scheduling is always a sensitive subject in hospital nursing units as well as most all volume-dependent areas. Regardless of the unit, finding a schedule that works for everyone and staffing perfectly to different volume levels is virtually an impossible task. Whether the organization uses a ratio-driven model or some form of acuity-based system, it will always appear that the unit is understaffed more often than not, but rarely will it be brought to management that there is a surplus of staff. There is no magic bullet for effective staffing, but if the issue is not addressed it can quickly lead to the most substantial source of waste in an organization. In order to address such a sensitive topic with cost saving measures, all stakeholders from department leaders to frontline caregivers must be included in an open dialogue. It all boils down to careful communication—establishing a reason or urgency for changing practice while acknowledging safe patient care as the most critical component to consider. It is about establishing a clear reason and respect for the change, and placing the accountability into the hands of those that do the work is without doubt the most effective tool. Successfully executing these types of large-scale changes does not require you to be a subject matter expert—rather a careful listener and motivator through solid communication skills.

Presently, I have a strong relationship with all nurse leaders in the organization, and have moved past initial clinical and experiential barriers to become a trusted adviser and advocate for the frontline caregivers. I certainly would not conclude that all clinical departments need a business-minded leader to work with the clinical staff, but it can without doubt be a wonderful partnership of mutual respect and benefit with the right department and individual.

As far as preparedness coming out of school, I believe any accredited program can offer all the tools you need to be successful in a fellowship or entry to mid-level management position. You should receive a diverse curriculum of finance, management theory, leadership courses, and the other basics, but more importantly it is the case studies, industry relationships, and the invaluable lessons of communication and professionalism that prepare you for the next step. I continue to be amazed with how many interns or fellows I have seen come out of various well-respected programs that simply disappoint. Professionalism in all phases, whether it be written communication, verbal, or formal presentations, goes a very long way. All of the practice with these skills may have seemed trivial to me during my undergraduate and graduate days, but they have proved far more valuable than the actual textbook course material.

A DAY IN THE LIFE OF A SENIOR VICE PRESIDENT FOR SYSTEM DEVELOPMENT AND CHIEF STRATEGY OFFICER

Tom Charles is the Senior Vice President for System Development and Chief Strategy Officer for Mount Nittany Health, State College, PA. Prior to joining Mount Nittany Health in February 2013, he served as Vice President for Strategic Planning for the Geisinger Health System, Danville, PA. Tom's 28-year career includes experience in behavioral health, hospital administration, ambulatory services management, strategic planning, clinical program and market development, and multi-specialty group practice management. Tom earned a BA in Psychology from Goshen College and MBA and MHA degrees from the University of Pittsburgh.

The role of a Chief Strategy Officer is shaped by the characteristics of the organization and the environment in which he or she works. Internal and external dynamics provide the backdrop and the framework for strategy development. A strategist needs to understand these dynamics and how they impact the organization's ability to act and succeed. The "days of my life" are a reflective of state of our organization, our opportunities, and our challenges.

Our health system is in the midst of transition from being "hospital-centric" to "system minded." Less than three years ago, the system acquired a large, well-established multi-specialty physician group, which has since grown to more than 100 providers.

Consequently, our system-mindedness, structures, and capabilities are still evolving. Our strategic plan is based on creating an integrated enterprise and leveraging these capabilities in our market and this forms the context for my work.

My days can best be described in four major buckets of work—listening/gathering, educating, planning, and tracking.

Listening/Gathering

A central part of my role is to understand the external and internal environments through data analytics and relationship building. The second aspect of this is probably the most important. Data without context is helpful, but limited. Context provides meaning and context is created through relationships.

Internal and external relationship building is essential. I spend a significant portion of my time meeting with system physicians, clinical, and administrative staff to learn about current performance, challenges, and opportunities. These conversations are vital to understanding our organizational capacities and competencies, where we excel and where we need to change. I try to balance this with similar interactions with leaders of partner and competitor organizations. My goal is to create relationships that facilitate the free exchange of information, which is essential to effective strategy.

Data analytics are also important for strategy formulation. Rarely a day passes that I do not review internal performance or financial analyses or access external data sources. Many of my meetings are organized around reviewing and disseminating this data to drive planning and monitor implementation.

Educating

It goes without saying that health care is a dynamic environment. As a strategist, part of my role is to help educate our Board, physicians, and staff about important dynamics that impact our future success. Along with the rest of our leadership team, I play an important role in ensuring our mission, vision, and strategic plan are well socialized across the organization.

I educate both directly and indirectly. It is common to find me delivering a presentation to our Board of Trustees, a meeting of our physician group leaders, a forum of hospital managers, or hospital staff. I believe face-to-face, two-way communication settings are critically important for building engagement and determining if your content is being delivered effectively. I also communicate indirectly through providing executive support for our Marketing and Communications team. I meet frequently with our Vice President for Marketing and Communications to discuss messaging as well as marketing and communication strategies, tactics, and implementation.

Planning

My planning activity spans a range from strategic planning work with our Executive Leadership and Board of Trustees to program planning with our physicians and clinical leadership.

In some aspects, planning is the most rewarding part of my daily work. Planning is a combination of tasks I enjoy—education, communication, and analysis. It is common to find me in meetings analyzing data and synthesizing internal and market information with our clinical and operational leadership. I especially enjoy the opportunity to work on multi-disciplinary clinical programs where we can combine our resources to deliver improved care and service to our community.

My strategic planning work takes place in Board meetings and retreats. Retreat settings are particularly valuable venues for relationship building, providing in-depth education about complex strategic issues, and decision making. Our Board of Trustees relies on our Executive Leadership team to ensure they are adequately educated and prepared to set us on the best strategic path. I work closely with our CEO to make sure we are effectively engaging the Board in this work.

Tracking

Strategies and plans do not matter if they are not implemented. A fourth component of my work is to ensure we are on track with execution. This happens in both formal and informal ways.

I work with our CEO to develop and track corporate and executive goals that tie to our strategic plan and ensure these goals are aligned across the Executive Leadership team. I also work with our Human Resources team to build and maintain a consistent goal alignment and tracking system across the organization. While each leader and manager is accountable for tracking and reporting their own progress and performance, part of my role is to ensure we have the systems in place to accomplish this in a systematic fashion.

On a more informal level, I allocate time to check in with leaders, managers, and front-line staff on the progress of key strategic initiatives. I believe this reinforces the importance of these projects to our overall strategic plan as well as encourages a level of accountability for results. These interactions also provide a three-dimensional context to the numbers and comments on tracking tools. Conversations reveal barriers—challenges that people are sometimes reluctant to commit to paper.

A day in my life is a rich mix of activities. I have the opportunity to stimulate dreams and ideas and to help them come to life. My work expands my horizons and understandings. Each day presents opportunity to impact people and our community in a positive way. It is rewarding to have that chance and to make the most of it.

A DAY IN THE LIFE OF AN INSURANCE EXECUTIVE

Cindy Helling serves as Select Health of South Carolina's executive director and has been employed by the company since its founding in 1995. She oversees the managed care company's operations throughout the state-wide service area. Ms. Helling has more than 20 years of experience in the health care industry, working for community hospitals and managed care organizations in Oklahoma, Florida, and South Carolina.

Select Health of South Carolina was the first to offer Medicaid managed care in our state in 1996. It was amazing to begin with nothing and create a health plan. In those early days as a start-up company, everyone pitched in on everything. There was never a concern about whose job it was to do XYZ. It just needed to be done. We all knew every member of our health plan and what their needs were, and we celebrated when the first baby was born to a mother on Select Health's First Choice plan.

During the first 12 years, Select Health's membership grew to 100,000, and in the 5 years after that, the number of members exploded to 270,000. Now, we welcome 1,200 babies to our plan each month. In fact, more than 80% of our members are aged 18 or younger. Despite the misconceptions about who receives Medicaid, these children and adolescents usually have parents who work, but at low-income levels.

Select Health has also grown to include 350 employees, or associates, as we like to say. Many work directly with our network of 8,000+ health care providers or with our members and their families, empowering them to understand and meet their health care needs. At Select Health, our mission is to help people get care, stay well, and build healthy communities. It is a mission we take to heart, one that motivates and energizes us, and we are fortunate to be part of the AmeriHealth Caritas Family of Companies, which is driven by the same goals.

An Early Start

I cannot say that I have a typical day as Select Health's executive director, because there are distinct roles that I play inside and outside our organization. I tend to many spinning plates, so to speak, and as Select Health grows, it seems the number of plates multiplies, too.

I usually start at 6 AM with business e-mail while I am still home. I use this as an opportunity to catch up and also respond to questions that I might have received the day before but wanted to consider more thoughtfully. This morning, I reviewed some purchase orders and contracts, and forwarded along an e-mail from the SC Department of Health and Human Services (SCDHHS) about a policy change that we must respond to within a week.

SCDHHS oversees the state's $6 billion Medicaid program, which is a competitive but controlled "marketplace." Those who qualify for Medicaid sign up to receive their benefits through one of several managed care plans, such as ours, which serves the most Medicaid recipients in the state.

While Select Health is not part of the government, we must respond rapidly to changes in government policies and regulations. Sometimes, these changes are out of our control, but we do our best to influence and encourage changes for the good of our members and others on Medicaid. Through the years, I have developed a positive rapport with people at all levels of the agency, including the legal staff, and the director of SCDHHS, who is on my speed dial.

Trust and Relationships

The truth is that I spend much of my time building relationships, not only with government leaders, but also health care providers and independent organizations, such as March of Dimes. Often, I go straight to a breakfast meeting before going to my office at the Select Health headquarters in the Charleston area. And it is not unusual for me to drive up to Columbia, our state capital, which is almost two hours away. Last week, I met with the medical director for the South Carolina Hospital Association. This week, I will meet twice with SCDHHS officials and travel to Columbia for a dinner honoring the Best Places to Work in South Carolina.

The fact that Select Health has received the Best Places to Work designation several times now speaks to our efforts to provide a nurturing, healthy workplace. This, in turn, has helped us keep many talented members of our workforce. We have a wonderful management team that has been in place for a long time. I know I can rely on them completely and trust in their decisions, and that allows me to be more effective as I multitask. There is no time for micromanaging if you are a leader in health care today.

I also strive to lead by example. Every time I step out of my office, I smile and show confidence, even if I am having a really crummy day. I want to be accessible, and recently held a series of town-hall style meetings with our associates. Each meeting lasted 30 minutes with me talking for 20 minutes and then opening up the floor for them. I warn that if they do not ask me questions, I will start asking them questions, and that gets a laugh and sparks the conversation. I try to hold these town hall meetings periodically and often wind up learning a great deal myself.

While I like to get away from the office for lunch, I usually eat out with colleagues, allowing us to take care of business in a relaxed environment. Much of my mornings and afternoons are filled with internal and external meetings. I prefer to talk face to face, and will occasionally travel to the AmeriHealth Caritas corporate office in Pennsylvania, so I can meet with the management there in person. When that is not possible, we try to videoconference.

Working Together

A key part of our success at Select Health has been our positive approach with providers. That includes physicians, pharmacists, urgent care facilities, community hospitals, and the Medical University of South Carolina, which has been an excellent partner for us.

I can relate to the provider perspective easily because I started my health care career as an information systems manager for community hospitals. When I switched to managed care, I quickly realized that when we team up with providers, value their opinions, and make the process as easy as possible for them, everyone wins, including our members. Because of this approach, we believe, providers are more likely to encourage their patients to choose First Choice by Select Health over our competitors.

We have found that prevention, education, and successful disease management pays off in terms of the health and quality of life of our members, and in terms of reduced spending. Within the past decade, Select Health has helped the state of South Carolina avoid $240 million in health care costs.

We also collaborate with other organizations to improve public health, and while there are many worthy causes, we try to choose those that best fit with our mission. For example, I serve on the board for the South Carolina March of Dimes, which is a great fit for Select Health, given the number of babies on our First Choice plan. In recent years, Select Health has worked with March of Dimes to stop unnecessary C-sections and early inductions and reduce the number of infant deaths, which remains a complex problem in our state.

Always Learning

I usually continue my workday until 6 PM unless I have a community function to attend. My role as a leader in public health requires that I be an effective communicator and coalition builder as well as a lifetime student, someone who is constantly studying, learning, and investigating. That is absolutely essential to anyone working with health care policy during this dynamic period of change. I love what I do, and I see the impact that we make in improving the quality of people's lives on a large scale.

A DAY IN THE LIFE OF A PHARMACEUTICAL SALES REPRESENTATIVE

Jessica Boss is a Senior Specialty Sales Consultant for Jazz Pharmaceuticals in Los Angeles, CA. Her product portfolio specializes in the psychiatry and mental health field in both inpatient and outpatient settings. Prior to working at Jazz, Jessica worked for Pfizer in the neuroscience and psychiatry business units where she represented eight different product brands over the course of seven years. Jessica finds motivation and joy each day in the knowledge that she is partnering with health care providers to help find the appropriate care and treatment for their patients.

Perhaps you have wondered what it was like to be a pharmaceutical sales representative. Maybe you have seen us stroll into your doctor's waiting room dressed in a nice suit bringing a full bag of sample prescription medications. Or possibly you have seen us portrayed in Hollywood movies and heard about the great "perks" such as a company car and lucrative starting salary. However, a career in pharmaceutical sales involves much more than sample drops and schmoozing with doctors; it is very much like running your own small business. You are given a defined sales territory along with a list of customers, marketing resources, expense budget, and a growth goal, and it is up to you to determine how to best utilize all those resources in such a way to reach or exceed your quota each year. Add in your competitor representatives also trying to achieve the same goals in the same market place, increasingly strict managed care reimbursements, competition from generic equivalents, new strict guidelines governing pharmaceutical interaction with customers, and an ever-changing health care market and you can start to get an idea of what makes this job so challenging and exciting.

Over the last 10 years, the industry has changed dramatically and therefore the skill set and job description of a pharmaceutical representative today is very different. Gone are the days of free tickets to sporting events and rounds of golf on the country's best courses. Today, a sales representative cannot even leave a pen or pad of paper with a product logo for a doctor due to increasing restrictions governing the interactions between health care providers and representatives. Your ability to make impact and drive sales therefore has to rely only on a representative's skill to be valued as a resource to the customer. The best representatives are those who truly understand their marketplace and business and can effectively strategize and align their own goals with the needs and wants of their customers in a compliant manner. Today's representatives are change agile, adaptable, self-motivated individuals who excel and thrive in a competitive ever-changing environment. They are experts in all things related to their therapeutic products, disease states, and managed care markets. And most importantly, they have an ability to make impact and standout among their competitors.

Getting the Job

Pharmaceutical Sales Representatives come from various backgrounds and college degrees. Some have had prior sales experience, others started in this field just out of college. However, what we all share in common is an ability to "sell" our past experiences and skill set during the interview process and demonstrate how we will be an asset to the company. If you cannot effectively sell yourself during the interview, why should the company believe you will be able to sell their product to a customer? A few important skills to highlight and be able to support with solid examples include self-motivation and organizational skills, an ability to learn complex information quickly and efficiently, communication and presentation skills, and an ability to interact and influence many different types of people and personalities. Linking these skill sets to how they will allow you to excel in this position will also demonstrate your basic understanding of selling skills 101—feature to benefit or need-based selling.

Networking within a pharmaceutical company can also potentially increase your odds of securing an interview and a job as a sales representative. Most companies value the opinion of their current employees and compensate them for new-hire recommendations that lead to a candidate being hired in an open position. Spending the day in the field with a representative will also offer you great insight into the position and usually translates well during the interview process to show initiative and a true understanding of the position. So do not be afraid to reach out to even distant contacts and express your interest. Sales Representatives are typically very social individuals with extroverted personalities who enjoy helping others. So practice your selling skills and "pitch" us why you would be a good fit for a career in pharmaceutical sales and "close" us on conducting a preceptorship ride-along in the field and passing along your résumé to HR.

Training

Before you even begin working with your physicians and other customers, most companies will have newly hired sales representatives complete an extensive training program to learn everything you will need to excel in this position. This typically includes courses and training modules in pharmacology, anatomy, specific disease states, competitive product profiles, clinical trials, managed care, and even selling skills. This time can be highly stressful on new representatives with multiple exams and tests as well as role playing and repetition to get you ready to be in the field in front of your customers. The goal is to provide a solid foundation and grow the confidence and skill set of new representatives.

A career in pharmaceutical sales involves continuous training and learning of new material. Throughout your career, you will regularly participate in learning and development programs to stay abreast on everything related to your current products, launch of new medications, changes in managed care, compliance guidelines for pharmaceutical representatives, and selling skills and strategy planning. Most companies will also bring all the representatives from a set region or the whole country together throughout the year to share ideas and best practices with each other. Because the field is constantly changing and evolving, sales representatives are continually learning and adapting. This is what keeps our job fun and never boring.

Day-to-Day Activities

A unique aspect to pharmaceutical sales selling versus other selling careers is the continuous relationship you are building with customers. There are rarely "cold calls" and your goal is to move the process forward instead of a "one-shot" chance to close a deal. Most physicians know and understand the general idea about your product or class of products but it is up to you to help them expand their knowledge of where and how to best utilize it. In order to be successful in this field, your ability to strategically plan will be essential. All of the tools will be handed to you: a customer base, marketing pieces, budget, and knowledge. It is up to the representative to take this information and then create a call routing schedule based on territory trends as well as health care providers' schedules and rules governing visitations and interactions with representatives. Restrategizing

each quarter depending on current success rates and changes to quota and company goals is also key to on-going success.

Once a representative has a call routing plan and strategic plan in place, it is time to execute on it each day. This starts with the pre-call plan. Each day, you begin by reviewing your plan for the day; what geography will you be covering that day, what appointments you have scheduled, who are the most important target accounts to see, etc. Then, before each interaction, or as the industry lingo refers to it, before each "call," with a physician, pharmacist, or hospital account, representatives review the current prescribing trends and create a goal or focus of discussion for that call. This can involve brainstorming some questions or information you wish to uncover that will move the sales process forward or a follow up item from a previous call.

Now it is time to visit your customer. During your interaction with the health care provider, you usually interact with a variety of different individuals, from the front office staff, to the nurse, to the billing manager, to the physician. Each one of these individuals is important and a good representative will "detail" or discuss product information with each stakeholder in the office. So often, office professionals outside of the physician can help influence your business even more so than the physician. The best representatives tend to follow a sales model that is focused on understanding the customer's needs first by asking effective open-ended questions and encouraging their customer to talk before pitching their product and finally asking for the business. In the old days of pharmaceutical selling, this used to be asking for a certain number of patients to be started on your product. Now, closing a customer involves encouraging them to think or try something different or new based on your conversation and proof offered to support doing so.

After each interaction with a customer, it is time to post-call plan and log your call. This involves taking note of what occurred during the interaction and any follow-up items that need to be addressed. If samples were left, it involves submitting the interaction to your company to keep a log of medication samples distributed. It is also a time of self-reflection. Did you meet your goal for the call as set in the pre-call plan? What could you do differently next time to reach your goal? How could you move the process forward to the next step? Now it is time to move on to the next customer and repeat the process all over again! At the end of each day, you log and submit all of your activities for the day to the company's mainframe. You also catch up on any e-mails and administrative items that need to be completed, such as expense reports or training initiatives and you plan and prepare for the following day's activities. While the basic nature of what representatives do day to day is repetitive, each day is far from monotonous due to the unique factor of working and interacting with so many different individuals throughout the day.

The Pros and Cons

There are days when I think that I have the best job in the world, I am able to run my own little business and interact with many different people each day ultimately helping health care providers better serve their patients. I drive a company car and can cruise around town between accounts with the windows down and radio on during nice days and am not confined to an office or cubicle from 9 to 5. I am able to combine my passion for health care and medicine with my outgoing chatty personality. Other days the reality of the challenges in this industry hit me hard. The need to always be "on" in front of customers, even when you are having a bad day, the need to be a chameleon to different offices, catering to multiple personalities all the time, even those you do not particularly like. In some cases, some offices treat representatives as simply a catering and sample drop service. There is always pressure to reach your quota each year and continually build upon your previous success. The solitary nature of the job and being on the road a lot on your own can be stressful. All of these things can make this job challenging. But at the end of each day, I can look back and be proud of the work I am doing, see the impact and influence I have

in my territory, and feel the progress moving forward to help more people. And that is why I love my career in pharmaceuticals.

Opinions contained here are solely Jessica Boss' and do not necessarily reflect the views of Jazz Pharmaceuticals.

A DAY IN THE LIFE OF A PRACTICE ADMINISTRATOR

Laura F. Leahy, MHA, is currently a practice manager of internal medicine and immediate care with Northwestern Memorial Physicians Group in Chicago, IL. She has also held practice management roles with Massachusetts General Hospital's department of radiology and Advocate Medical Group's general surgery practice. Laura has a passion for optimizing operations through process improvement and creating mechanisms to care for underserved populations.

Practice administrators, or practice managers, are responsible for managing one or multiple physician office locations, typically within a larger medical group. They are leaders in their practices and are responsible for managing the daily operations of their practice areas as well as developing, planning, overseeing, and implementing new processes per organizational standards. Practice managers typically operate in outpatient, ambulatory, or primary care practices.

A practice manager's day is rarely planned, as it is subject to change based on the needs of the practice. In addition to managing the day-to-day operations, a practice manager is responsible for finding ways to expand and improve their business to meet patient and organizational needs. They must be well versed in all aspects of medical group operations, including revenue cycle, insurance, quality, scheduling, registration, referrals, information systems, and process improvement. Additionally, they must stay apprised of changing trends in health care delivery systems, payment systems, and industry standards. This is key for practices to remain competitive while preparing for the future of health care delivery.

The most basic functions in a typical day include ensuring staffing needs are met, addressing patient issues, handling provider needs, and holding to high standards of clinical quality. Mid-level functions include managing budgets, productivity, staffing variances, and patient satisfaction for the office. Each of these requires strategic communication with key stakeholders, including providers, staff, and executive leadership. A practice administrator must also work on long-term organizational projects such as utilizing process improvement methods to decrease expenses while increasing quality and access, implementing new service lines, and creating business development strategies to drive volume to the practice.

As with other leaders in health care management, a practice administrator's role has changed over the past few years. Increased focus on primary and preventive care now means that practice managers must collaborate with other health care entities to provide the highest quality of care at a lower cost as a medical home.

In short, a practice administrator's job is highly dynamic and always subject to change. A practice administrator must have the discipline to handle the immediate needs, manage the intermediate needs, and plan for the long-term and often unknown landscape.

Because the day of a practice administrator can vary, please see two actual examples below.

Day 1

The manager gets a call in the morning from a medical assistant stating they are unable to come in for the day due to an illness. The assistant's provider has a full schedule, so the practice manager immediately leaves for the office to rearrange staffing. The new staffing model is assigned and communicated to providers and staff members.

Next, the practice manager has to handle a patient complaint. A patient was seen at the office for an ankle sprain while she is six weeks pregnant. The patient was given a referral for an x-ray, as the provider thought the radiology suite would have appropriate equipment to shield the embryo. When the patient arrived at the imaging center, she was told she could not have the x-ray because of the potential danger it presented to her pregnancy. Upon hearing this, the patient called the practice manager furious that the provider had recommended a course of treatment that had potential to endanger her pregnancy. The practice manager spends the next hour gathering information about the case, collaborating with the patient satisfaction manager, and creating a plan to appease the patient. She then calls the patient, listens to the patient's concerns, and presents her strategy to help the patient overcome this experience.

Once the patient has been appropriately appeased, the practice manager completes afternoon rounds. During the rounds, she notices that some sharps containers are full, the lab inventory is low, and that patient confidentiality was violated outside one of the offices. The practice manager documents these occurrences and sits down with employees to take corrective action on the urgent items. She adds the other items to her agendas for staff meetings.

Next, that practice manager has a regular call with her director. The practice locations are at various sites in the community and therefore, the practice manager utilizes an autonomous management approach. The director and manager review the clinical indicators, financial statements, and productivity for the medical practice. For any indicator that does not meet its budget, the manager presents a brief action plan. This may include business development ideas to drive volume, process improvement ideas to reduce waste, or new processes to improve quality. They also discuss any staff issues, provider needs, and general clinic needs.

At this point, the practice manager attends a meeting to improve patient access across the entire medical group. The project's goal is to increase the patient satisfaction score around a patient's ability to access the clinic. This project involves input from various departments, including the call center, information systems, operations, business development, and revenue cycle. At the conclusion of this meeting, the practice manager briefly meets with other practice managers to discuss challenges with a new consent form that has been mandated.

Finally, the practice manager checks in with the site before departing for the day. After rounding with the staff and providers, she leaves with her pager in hand, ready to be contacted with any issues that arise.

Day 2

The practice manager arrives at the clinic to find that the early morning provider is running 20 minutes behind schedule. Patients in the waiting area are angry and becoming inpatient. The practice manager immediately investigates the reason for the provider running behind schedule. Once the cause is determined, the practice manager works with the provider and their assistant to rectify the situation. Patients who are waiting are notified of the estimated time at which they will be seen, are offered alternative appointments, and/or service recovery items.

Immediately following this, the practice manager has a conference call with a team that is working on opening a new practice location. The team meets for one hour to review the project plan while each member provides his or her respective updates. The call includes updates on construction progress, workflow design, marketing strategies, business development plans, provider schedules, and staffing needs.

At the conclusion of that call, the manager has another call with a vendor that is piloting a new scheduling system at the manager's location. They discuss the pilot's progress and noted deficiencies in the application. Thinking to the future, they brainstorm potential challenges and finally outline tasks to be completed before the next week's call.

Next, the practice manager has a lunch meeting with providers where they discuss challenges associated with the implementation of new radiology and cardiology order sets. The practice manager clarifies some confusion by restating the importance of using the new order sets instead of relying on a referral

team to place and track the order. Additionally, the practice manager redemonstrates how providers should be utilizing the new order sets. The providers demonstrate proficiency in utilizing the new system while the manager addresses any lingering concerns.

After the lunch meeting, the practice manager has a meeting with the billing manager. They discuss the practice's progress in increasing the dollar amount of past due balances collected at time of service, proper coding practices, and strategies to reduce the number of patients who are sent to collections for past due balances. Next, they discuss long-term trends and visualize a future where the same services receive less reimbursement while coping with increased expenses.

At this point, the practice manager returns to her office to focus on making progress on the projects that have been discussed during the day. A brief interruption occurs when a staff member asks for vacation and has to be denied due to staffing needs. An additional break occurs when the patient communication portal goes down and the front desk requires additional assistance to handle the influx of phone calls. After that, the manager spends the rest of the day working on projects.

What do these scenarios have in common? They both demand that the practice manager juggle multiple short- and long-term priorities in a timely manner. They require precise triage skills, a high degree of flexibility, and an intimate understanding of the clinic's operations. These duties necessitate an ability to act autonomously, drive change, collaborate with stakeholders, communicate effectively, and understand the complex and ever-changing health care landscape.

Practice managers are always busy; are not afraid to get their hands dirty; are sensitive to the needs of patients, staff, and providers; and genuinely care about providing great care to patients. They are constantly collaborating and communicating, redesigning and improving, assessing and developing; all for the sake of providing the best care at the best value to their patients. In summary, they are master jugglers balancing practice, organizational, and industry needs.

A DAY IN THE LIFE OF A HEALTH CARE-RELATED PROFESSIONAL ASSOCIATION EXECUTIVE

Diane Simmons, MPA, RN, CAE, is vice president of education and certification for the Healthcare Financial Management Association (HFMA). Prior to joining HFMA, Diane was the CEO of a health care certification consortium and also served as Executive Director for a number of specialty nursing associations within an association management company. As a health care professional, Diane served in a number of roles from clinical nursing to hospital administration. Diane earned a BSN from Montana State University and a MPA from Seattle University.

As the Vice President for Education and Certification, I oversee the development and implementation of a wide range of educational products targeted at a diverse group of learners in a number of different formats for the Healthcare Financial Management Association (HFMA). HFMA is a professional membership association serving around 40,000 members working in a variety of roles within the health care industry. The primary practice setting for health care finance professionals is a hospital or health care system with titles ranging from Chief Financial Officer to staff accountant. There is diversity of role, practice setting, and career stage.

HFMA has two primary components to its learning portfolio—event-based learning and digital learning. Event-based learning programs are traditional conferences, courses, and seminars. Basically, any event in which there is a live instructor with coffee service at the breaks. Digital learning formats include webinars, a virtual conference, and online learning. All of the education delivered through HFMA meets standards defined by the CE provider, the National Association of State Boards of Accountancy. We set a high priority on quality and attendee satisfaction. We conduct formal and informal research on attendee satisfaction and use that feedback to modify or amplify programs.

Coordinating the development of an education program takes an entire village—most often it feels like a small city. The activities for any program range from topic selection relevant to the industry, instructional design, format development, marketing, logistics management, technology assessment, speaker management, registration processing, vendor alignment, and attendee engagement just to name a few. While the professional development team is comprised of 10 individuals, at any point in time 40 or more people from other disciplines and departments may work on a particular program. The planning process for a large meeting, such as our annual convention is at least a 16-month process. As I write this piece, we are now eight months away from the annual conference. Today, I signed the final contract with a speaker bureau for the last of our three keynote speakers, reviewed and confirmed the marketing plan, provided feedback on the new format design, had a conference call with a board member about a session she will lead, and met with a team member to revise the convention center contract to expand the allocated space. Oftentimes, the level of detail required is excruciatingly painful. However, managing the details ensures that the event is an educationally enriching and engaging experience for those who attend. After all, if a detail such as coffee service is missed in the process, we know that there will be many unhappy folks especially at an early riser session at 7 AM. Because of the extraordinary amount of work that goes into the planning and preparation of a large conference, it can appear effortless to those who attend. However, I liken it to ice skating—as a novice it looks easy until you actually step on the ice. As you pick yourself up for the 10th time, you develop an appreciation for the years of practice and preparation that go into making Olympians appear effortless as they glide over the ice.

HFMA's professional certification program has been in place for many years and is intended to define the standards of practice expected by professionals with several years' experience in health care business or finance. There is a rigorous exam process overseen by a volunteer Board of Examiners comprised by experts in variety of roles within the industry. In addition to the professional certification program, we also administer an entry-level certification program and have several newly developed technical certification products. Today, I met with the director for that program and approved a final contract with our testing vendor, reviewed the agenda for the upcoming board meeting, and discussed a new plan for delivery of the certification program. Based on our strategic positioning work at the executive level, I want to make sure our programs are aligned with that vision.

So how do I really spend my time? My role is responsible not only for the oversight and management of the education and certification functions, but I am also involved at the strategic level with our executive team and board of directors to identify trends in the industry and to facilitate matching educational resources in response to those shifting trends. These past couple of years has been particularly challenging and rewarding as we have attempted to provide real-time education to our members in a rapidly changing environment. Here is an example of how we responded to the Supreme Court Decision on the individual mandate. We knew in advance there were three scenarios that were possible outcomes of the decision. I pulled together our internal technical experts and we mapped out those possible scenarios. If it were struck down, what implications would that have for the industry? If it were upheld, what impact might that have? We fully developed the content plan for each of the three scenarios in advance. The speech writers then took the content and developed three separate presentations. We engaged our webinar platform for three potential dates we thought were likely post announcement. Because of the expected volume on the call, we had to purchase additional capacity on the platform. Marketing messages to be delivered in an electronic format were prepared, again for three possible scenarios and three potential dates. Speakers were put on the ready for each of the scenarios. The Business Development team secured a vendor sponsor for the webinar and the registration processing was prepared in advance. Once the announcement was made, we were fully prepared with a date, time, speakers, con-

tent, and messaging that was delivered within five days of the announcement. To those participating on the call, it appeared flawless and was a "just-in-time" learning experience. If we had not prepared well in advance, I can assure you it wouldn't have happened in real time, and would likely have had more than a few glitches. We provided a valuable education experience to our members that reinforced the value of belonging to HFMA.

In addition to the program development aspects of our educational portfolio, I also have accountability for operations management of our entire education portfolio. Revenue comes from registration fees and vendor support. Expenses include everything from audiovisual equipment rental, speaker support, travel, hotel rental, marketing, and yes . . . coffee service. Monthly, I review progress on financial performance of key program areas and am prepared to shift resources if needed, make the hard call on program elements that may not be performing well and my favorite part—celebrate success!

I wish I could define a logical career path that led me to this role. I am a proud member of the nursing profession. In my early clinical career, I enjoyed learning and at one point was thrust into a teaching role as a volunteer leader in my profession. I earned a Master's degree in Public Administration and spent many years in administrative roles in a health care system. I have always been active in my profession as a volunteer leader, program faculty, and board advisor. Several years ago, I moved into a staff role within a professional association and have held several roles within the association world all devoted to health care. While there is not a defined career path in my story, there were some clear decision points along the way. First, I fell in love with nursing and found that I was more effective as an advocate and leader than as a bedside nurse. Know your strengths. I got involved in my professional association as a way to figure out what I needed to do to be more effective. The unintended consequence of that decision was not only did I learn to improve my practice, but I met people and gathered resources that would open doors for me along the way. I also learned that when opportunities arise that will take you out of your comfort zone, do not hesitate, just do it. Public speaking, writing for publication, and developing strategic plans were never on my "wanna do" list. Stay open to the possibilities.

What I love about what I do is that I get to work with the best and the brightest every day in an industry that I am passionate about and am able to help effect change at a strategic level. And yes, part of that is making sure there is enough hot coffee to keep learning real.

A DAY IN THE LIFE OF A TECHNOLOGY EXECUTIVE

Steven Wagman is vice president for Enterprise Solutions Implementation at Siemens Medical Solutions, USA, based in Malvern, Pennsylvania. He brings 30 years of experience in health care consulting, implementation, and support services for health care information systems, diagnostic medical imaging, and the digital integrated health system. The Siemens Healthcare Sector is one of the world's largest suppliers to the health care industry and a trendsetter in medical imaging, laboratory diagnostics, medical information technology, and hearing aids. Siemens Health Care employs approximately 51,000 employees worldwide.

Working in the health care industry is a privilege. As such, I begin each day with the end in mind. The patient lying in the hospital bed, on the operating room table, or in the MRI scanner is somebody's parent, child, sibling, relative, or friend. Keeping this in mind keeps me focused and grounded in everything I do and how I conduct my business.

My interest in health care started at an early age, although it took different twists and turns; from aspiring to be a physical therapist to sports medicine and finally a college major in Health Planning and Administration, with a pre-professional emphasis. Early in my college career, however, I realized that medical school was probably not in the cards for

me so my focus became learning as much about the United States and comparative health care systems as I could absorb.

My internship experience, which took place at a small, long-term care children's hospital, associated with a large urban acute care facility, was invaluable to me in developing a practical understanding of the patient care process, how care providers interacted with patients and their families and the nuances of working through the various health care processes that you do not read about in textbooks. One of the projects I worked on during that internship, keeping in mind that this was before today's electronic health record systems (EHRs), required me to sift through hundreds of paper medical records looking for discreet data elements to support grant applications. Little did I know that this experience would be the basis for my initial assignment in my first "paid" professional position. This is an important lesson in the value that an internship provides to a student, although it may not be realized until later.

Upon graduation, I've spent my 30-year career in health care IT consulting, Radiology/PACS, and medical imaging in a variety of consultative, managerial, and executive roles. This career path has afforded me the opportunity to work in hundreds of hospitals and health care provider organizations, including physician practices, urban hospitals, critical access hospitals, facilities that are part of for-profit hospital chains, diagnostic imaging centers, etc. In my own way, I can support the patient care process and never have a scalpel in my hand (which is good news for the patient).

The technology and innovation in medical imaging is fascinating, not in a "technology for the sake of technology" way, but rather for what the technology can do in a practical application.

For example, when I was in school, the term *exploratory surgery* was common (if in doubt, just watch reruns of any medical television show from the 1970s or 1980s).Today, we do not hear that term very often because we can now use imaging technology to see soft tissue, blood vessels, and organs inside the human body to diagnose disease, instead of cutting the patient open, as well as its use during treatment. In many respects, medical imaging has become a standard of care, resulting in less pain, shorter hospital stays (or to avoid a hospital stay), and reduced time lost from work.

Working with health care providers to insure that they have the proper tools to diagnose and treat disease, understanding everything from their business service lines to the physical facilities and environmental systems required to support the technology, the patient experience and the clinical care giver is what I (or my staff) provides each day.

One of the most profound experiences that I have had was visiting a customer (a surgeon and radiologist) several years ago, who described a recent case and their use of a new surgical suite, which we helped them plan, and included our MRI technology to visualize and pinpoint the brain tumor in a nine-year-old child; plan the surgery, and while in the surgical suite slide the patient back into the MRI to insure that they excised the entire tumor prior to closing the skull and completing the surgical procedure.

They showed me the images taken pre- and post-op and explained that prior to the availability of this surgical suite, they would plan and perform the surgery, sparing as much normal brain tissue as possible, but wanting to remove the entire tumor to avoid a reoccurrence later requiring additional surgery. If you are a parent and see, hear, and feel the passion as the doctors described this (with visuals), how can you not be personally affected by this story, especially when you see the photograph of this now healthy little girl?

Now, professionally, we all have our skills and areas for continued development over the course of our careers. After 30 years in health care, I find that the pace of my learning continues to increase. I maintain that the most important attribute that you obtain in college is the ability to think broadly and learn how to learn.

During the course of my career, I have spent the majority of my years in "road warrior" positions,

meaning that my week consisted of Monday through Friday travel, either by car or by plane, depending on the geography that I had responsibility for at the time. Over the past several years, my travel has included international destinations, which has also afforded me the opportunity to learn more about the health systems in other countries, again, from a practical standpoint in speaking with colleagues and visiting facilities; both from a patient care perspective as well as how health care is financed and how limited capital resources are deployed.

I have also relocated twice during my career. I have found that between the travel and two relocations (not to mention 60–70 hour work weeks); bearing some of the burden, and certainly contributing to my professional success was the support that my wife provided, especially as we raised two children (one with special needs).

I always coach my employees about staying relevant, and that dinosaurs became extinct for a reason, so I always encourage continued development (theirs and mine) and not allowing myself to becoming a dinosaur. What I mean by this is that the health care regulations and laws change over time; technology and its applications change too (generally more rapidly than regulations and payment systems). Embracing change and staying ahead of the learning curve is a business imperative.

On a personal basis, I work toward long-term professional relationships that become friendships over time. Colleagues and customers that I started my career with 30 years ago are many of the same people I still speak with and work with today, although they may be scattered elsewhere across the industry. Relationship building, networking, and conducting myself with the highest degree of honesty and integrity is an absolute requirement in the professional work world.

In working with customers and colleagues; maintaining an even keel, a good attitude, and following through on what I say and commit to, are some of the key attributes that I work hard to maintain. A good attitude means taking the initiative, being willing to help a customer, or colleague beyond what is "required" and insuring that my work product is of the highest quality. It is all about building trust and creating value, for an employee, a customer or colleague.

When someone asks what I do in my day-to-day responsibilities, I tell them that I create the opportunity to match my customers' (or employee) business or personal need with the capabilities that I can bring to the table. It is not just about a product or service; it is about creating value and solving a business problem.

Again, keeping the end in mind, it is about the patient and I have been privileged to work in health care for the last 30 years.

Note: Any statements and opinions are mine alone and does not necessarily represent those of Siemens Healthcare.